# ENDORSEMENTS

AWESOME!!! Wish Fibromyalgia came with an instruction manual? Now it does! In her outstanding book, Kelly Hemingway RN turns the complex into straight forward. Having been there herself, she offers the best of spiritual, psychological and medical guidance so you can begin the journey to Get Well NOW!

*Jacob Teitelbaum MD*

Author of *From Fatigued to Fantastic!*
and *The Fatigue and Fibromyalgia Solution*

When I embarked on the journey of applying for Social Security Disability in February 2016, I did so with a tremendous amount of trepidation after reading and hearing the horror stories of so many that had come before me. It was then that I came across Kelly Hemingway. She had posted some information on a Facebook support group page that immediately piqued my interest. I reached out to her for further information. It was then that she 'gifted' me with the valuable resources and advise that she had. I did not know the value of these until May 2016 when to my utter amazement I was APPROVED for SSDI a mere three months after applying! I truly believe that after reading over the information that she has accumulated through her own research was I successful. I am grateful for the peace of mind she has aided me in attaining! Thank you from the bottom of my heart Kelly!

Just one word—AWESOME!!!

*Monica H. Mullins*

# FIBROMYALGIA:
## HOPE BEYOND THE PAIN

KELLY HEMINGWAY, RN, MSN

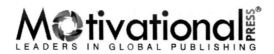

Published by Motivational Press, Inc.
1777 Aurora Road
Melbourne, Florida, 32935
www.MotivationalPress.com

Manufactured in the United States of America.

ISBN:  978-1-62865-312-0

# CONTENTS

## CHAPTER 6

## CHAPTER 7

## CHAPTER 8

## RESOURCES

*I'd like to dedicate this book to my husband Dave, my daughter Katie, my 2 dads, and my best friend Laurie Saunders. Without their love, ongoing support, and encouragement this book would have never been possible.*

## FOREWORD

---

# DON'T LEARN TO LIVE WITH IT!

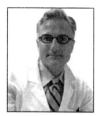 I'm so excited about this book! We need this book. You need this book. There are so many wonderful tips, suggestions, and must know information in this book, you'll quickly have multiple pages colored in highlighter ink.

Thankfully, this is not another doom and gloom book, advocating how to "learn to live with fibromyalgia." It is a book filled with cutting edge, information for overcoming fibromyalgia.

Too many of those with fibromyalgia have been led to believe by doctors, friends, and even loved ones, that they are either lazy, crazy or simply a hypochondriac.

And unfortunately, conventional medicine has pretty much given up on fibromyalgia. Most doctors, if they believe fibromyalgia exists, and many still don't, have come to the erroneous belief, that once you get fibromyalgia, you'll have it for life, and, there's nothing you can do about it. Their goal is just to help you manage it. They'll recommend an assortment of different medications to treat the ever-growing list of fibromyalgia symptoms. A drug to put you to sleep, a drug to wake you up, drugs for pain, low moods, irritable bowel, restless legs, and on, and on it goes.

They will tell you to "learn to live with it."

Many of my patients when they first start working with me, are on half a dozen to a dozen drugs. The problem is you don't know which drugs, if any, are actually helping. How would you? You have good days and bad days, no matter how many drugs you are taking. So who knows? Some drugs have side effects that are causing more symptoms, symptoms that mimic those of fibromyalgia-fibro fog, bloating, gas, low moods, poor sleep, pain, etc.

I'm not anti-drug; I'm really not, because there's definitely a time and a place for drug therapy. When I'm working with my patients, I'm a realist and if they need medications, so be it. But no one has a drug deficiency. The only way to feel good again, and stay that way, is to get healthy. Drugs don't make you healthy. They can be helpful, but they don't make you healthy. Long term, they are a dead end.

The drugs for fibromyalgia may or may not, reduce the symptoms, but long term they don't work, often create more problems, and most always compromise one's vitality. A collection of weapons

Conventional doctors who treat fibromyalgia patients know this. They know they have nothing in their arsenal that will help their patients, at least long term. Managing the symptoms is all they can do. **Finding And Fixing The Causes Of Fibromyalgia Symptoms Is The Key To Getting Healthy And Feeling Good Again.**

Fibromyalgia is just a name of a syndrome that has common symptoms associated with the syndrome. It's a name-it doesn't cause anything! There are underlying causes for the low energy, chronic pain, poor sleep, brain fog, and other symptoms/warning signs, associated with fibromyalgia. Finding and fixing these causes, with functional medicine, is the key to getting healthy and feeling good again.

## FUNCTIONAL MEDICINE

Functional medicine addresses the underlying causes of disease, using a systems-oriented approach and engaging both patient and practitioner in a therapeutic partnership. It is an evolution in the practice of medicine that better addresses the healthcare needs of the 21st century. By shifting the traditional disease-centered focus of medical practice to a more patient-centered approach, functional medicine addresses the whole person, not just an isolated set of symptoms. Doctors who practice functional medicine seek to find and fix causes, not merely treat symptoms. Covering up symptoms with drugs often leads to more health problems.

After two decades of treating fibromyalgia patients, I've come to the realization and I learned this the hard way, the only way to feel good again, and have the opportunity to actually stay feeling good, is you have to get healthy.

It's not about "learning to live with it," it is about finding and fixing the underlying causes of your fibromyalgia symptoms. It is about getting healthy and staying healthy!

Kelly's book is big step in the right direction for getting and staying healthy. You can feel good again. It takes hard work, and often the right health coach/doctor, but it can be done. Kelly and thousands of my patients are getting healthy, feeling good again, and not learning to live with fibromyalgia. So can you.

Rodger Murphree D.C., C.N.S

www.treatingandbeating.com

Author of: _Treating and Beating Fibromyalgia_ and _Chronic Fatigue Syndrome Heart Disease What Your Doctor Won't Tell You_

Check out my fibromyalgia blog at www.thefibrodoctor.co-

# Chapter 1

## FIBRO: FACT OR FICTION

### A Letter From Fibromyalgia

Dear Miserable Human Being,

Hi, my name is Fibromyalgia, and I'm an invisible chronic illness. I am now 'velcroed' to you for life. Others around you can't see me or hear me, but YOUR body feels me. I can attack you anywhere and anyway I please. I can cause severe pain, or if I am in a good mood, I can just cause you to ache all over. Remember when you and Energy ran around together and had fun? I took Energy from you and gave you Exhaustion. Just try to have fun now! I also took Good Sleep from you and in its place gave you Fibro Fog (a.k.a.) Brain Fog. I can make you tremble internally or feel cold or hot when everyone else feels normal. Oh yeah, I can make you feel anxious or depressed too. If you have something planned, or are looking forward to a great day, I can take that away too. You didn't ask for me. I chose you for various reasons: that virus you had that you never quite recovered from, that car accident, childbirth, the death of a loved one, or maybe it was those years of abuse and trauma. Well, anyway, I'm here to stay! I hear you're going to see a doctor who can get rid of me. I'm 'ROFL' (rolling on the floor laughing)! Just try! You will have to go to many, many doctors until you find one who can help you effectively. In fact, you'll see many doctors who tell you 'it's all in your head' (or some version of that). If you do find a doctor willing to treat this 'non-disease', you will be put on pain pills, sleeping pills, and energy pills. You will be told you are suffering from anxiety or depression, given a TENS unit, told if you just sleep and exercise properly, I will go away. You'll be told to think positively, poked, prodded, and most of all, you will not be taken seriously when you cry to the doctor how debilitating life is for you every single day! Your family, friends, and coworkers will all listen to you until they just get tired of hearing about how I make you feel, and that I'm a debilitating disease. Some of them will say things like "Oh, you're just having a bad day", or "Well, remember, you can't expect to do the things you used to do 20 years ago," not hearing that you said "20 DAYS ago"! Some will just start talking behind your back, while you slowly feel that you are losing your dignity, trying to make them understand, especially when you are in the middle of a conversation with a 'normal' person, and can't remember what you were going to say next!

In closing, you've probably figured out that the ONLY place you will get any real support and understanding in dealing with me is with Other People with Fibromyalgia! They are the only ones who will understand your complaints of unrelenting pain, insomnia, fibro fog, the inability to perform the everyday tasks that 'normal people' take for granted. Remember, I'm stuck to you like Velcro – and I expect we'll be together for the rest of your life.

Have a nice day!!

Author is unknown.

## PERSONAL JOURNEY

*"Face reality as it is, not as it was,
or as you wish it to be."*

~Jack Welch

You have to help me. With tears welled up in my eyes, I pleaded with my health practitioner. My body hurts everywhere. It felt like every square inch of me was covered in bruises. It hurt for my daughter or husband to even touch my skin. I had some particular spots that hurt worse than others including in my neck, over my shoulder blades, and down both sides of my spine and down to my knees. The fatigue that accompanied the pain made me feel I could sleep for weeks.

It had only been a few weeks since I suffered from an almost fatal severe allergic reaction to an antibiotic I was taking for bronchitis. I spent a few days before Christmas in the hospital but made it home in time for the holidays. I was physically present, but mentally, I was lost in a far-a-way land.

I followed up with my practitioner a couple weeks later and she sent me for blood draws. The only lab that came back positive showed I had generalized inflammation. So the next several months were a myriad of referrals to every single kind of specialist imaginable. The allergist had no idea why I had hives, scratched his head, and referred me to the University of Michigan. The doctors there told me there that I was under too much stress and I had acid reflux which was eating my vocal cords. They prescribed me 300 mg of Zantac twice a day and told me to take stress management classes. I left that building feeling like I could spit bullets.

Oh my God in heaven, am I crazy? I asked my husband if he thought I was nuts. He assured me that was not the case and that we would have to continue on our journey to find the right doctor. I buried my face in my hands and cried. The right doctor didn't exist for me. It hurt to walk. I had the following signs and symptoms that nobody could diagnose: deep constant muscle aches all over, inability to sleep, pain in arm joints, legs, ankles, muscle weakness, unsteady balance, and a red sunburned skin rash located on my arms and chest.

After another visit with my nurse practitioner, I mentioned the possibility of fibromyalgia. This idea came from my mother-in-law who had a friend who was a doctor. Patty's eyes lit up and said; Oh my, YES! I think that's exactly what it is. She applied pressure to certain areas of my body which caused me severe pain, then told me I certainly had enough 'tender points' and other symptoms to convince her that it was fibromyalgia. She started me on medication that same day, but advised me it might be awhile before I feel the effects of the medicine. Could this be the right diagnosis? I was not even sure it was a real condition. Did my practitioner grab at that diagnosis because she couldn't figure anything else out? I was not so convinced I had fibro, but happy to have something I could hold onto as a diagnosis as opposed to being crazy.

I was still experiencing odd signs and symptoms such as a sunburn rash on my face, neck, upper shoulders and back, foggy thinking among many other issues, so my journey of seeing specialists continued. The next doctor I saw was a rheumatologist. Oh glorious day, I thought I finally found a doctor who was going to dig me out of the ditch, give me my life back, and explain all my other odd symptoms that were interfering with my ability to function. He was younger and on the cutting edge of knowledge. He called the rash on my chest and back a "shall rash" because it looks like one is wearing a shawl. He thought he found a diagnosis of dermatomyositis and ordered another myriad of tests including a muscle biopsy on my upper thigh. It seemed I fit the perfect profile for this very rare condition. Finally, maybe an answer. Then my world came crashing down. The biopsy was negative and the doctor basically said, you are back to square one. Go back to your primary doctor and start over, there's nothing more I can do for you. I was devastated.

Upon arriving home that night, I was pretty convinced I needed to be admitted to the psych ward. I was sad and depressed. Anxiety filled my mind wondering if anyone would ever find anything wrong with me or if I would have to live the rest of my life feeling half dead.

I was trying with all my might to continue working as the Licensed Practical Nursing (LPN) coordinator of a community college. I took my students to a clinical setting and took my nebulizer because I was wheezing so badly. I had my students take turns giving me breathing treatments and told them it was a good learning experience, and it was. Little did I know I was driving myself further into the ground of denial by trying to continue working.

Throughout the time I tried to work, I was hospitalized a multitude of times for what they called adrenal insufficiency. Doctors told me that my adrenal glands were not working right. Then I was admitted for asthma, and again for adrenal insufficiency because my body would not let me get off steroids. When you take a steroid by mouth the adrenal glands, which normally make steroids, get lazy. So in essence, mine were on vacation. However, I had a fantastic endocrinologist I had worked with for many years in the hospital, who was consulted to help my case. He had worked at the Mayo clinic and told me that is where I belonged. It took some work, but I finally got to Mayo clinic.

I was so excited as my husband and I sat on the plane on our way to Mayo Clinic in Rochester MN. Looking out the windows into the clouds, I was hopeful for the first time in a long time. My thoughts were that I was going to get in, see the best specialists in the world, and go home all better. I just knew I was finally going to get answers. After all, they were among the most reputable facilities one could get to. However, my spirit was soon to be crushed. Over the next few days I saw a multitude of specialists who simply said they just didn't know what was wrong. I had blood tests, chest x-rays, pulmonary function tests, echocardiograms, and even a 24 hour urine collection that I had to carry around in my lap as my husband wheeled me around in a wheelchair because I was too short of breath to walk.

On my fourth and final visit to Mayo Clinic I saw a very young looking professional neurologist who was the only compassionate doctor I had while I was there. I asked her if she had any idea what was wrong with me because I didn't believe that I had fibromyalgia. She spoke softly and said to me, "Kelly, I have reviewed all your medical files extensively and I firmly believe that you do have fibromyalgia." There are most likely other underlying conditions that could be masked by the fact that you are on steroids, but I want you to go down to our educational clinic and see a fibro counselor. Can you do that? I gulped and told her yes as long as they could get us in soon because we had a plane to catch that afternoon.

Prior to getting to the fibro counselor, I had my final consultation with a doctor who was supposed to wrap all the information, labs, and test results into a neat package and give me a diagnosis and treatment recommendations. My heart was pounding; my heart sank into my stomach. I could tell by the look on his face that it wasn't good news. The next words he said caused me to run from the room crying uncontrollably. I am sorry Kelly, but we cannot come up with an answer for any of your peculiar symptoms with the exception of fibromyalgia.

So that's it; I walked away with a diagnosis of fibromyalgia feeling like death warmed over. As if that was not bad enough, I soon found myself in a cool, plain, and un-inviting board room for fibromyalgia education. Sitting across from me and my husband was a fibro counselor and I could tell by the glaring look on her face, she meant business.

She pulled no punches and spoke these words that are still seared into my brain, "Kelly, your life as you know it is over." It felt as if someone had slapped me in the face then punched me in the gut as she spoke those gut wrenching words. She continued, "Your life will never be the same." I put my head down on the table and burst out crying uncontrollably. My husband placed his hand on my back and tried to comfort me, but there was no comfort found. I felt empty, sad, and despondent. It felt as if someone had ripped the rug from under my feet and I found myself suddenly on the floor with no way to get up.

As the educator handed me booklets and pamphlets and discussed ways my life would have to be modified, I decided that I was not going to believe this was real. I grabbed the booklets through tear filled eyes and told the lady we had a plane to catch.

Walking out of that office in 2011, in my stubborn spirit, I was determined to prove that there was some kind of a mistake. My plan was to go back to Michigan and proceed onward with my career as a nursing instructor just as I had before the last of my four trips to Mayo clinic which were all but a waste of time! They put me through almost every kind of imaginable test that invaded, electrified, and assaulted my physical body. I was done. I had enough and was taking my life back......
or so I thought.

## Is Fibro Real?

In a word: YES! Fibromyalgia is real. The first thing I want to emphasize to all of you suffering out there is to know that "YOU ARE NOT ALONE." Even though there is so much information yet to be discovered about Fibromyalgia Syndrome (FMS), there is a lot of evidence that has been discovered to help you cope and survive from one day to the next. Since FMS is not a cookie cutter illness, meaning it does not affect any same two patients in the same way, one of the keys to getting proper care is to educate yourself. That is one of the primary reasons I am writing this book-to educate patients, families, and healthcare professionals. Another reason is to legitimize and provide proof that FMS is real.

Fibromyalgia is a collection of symptoms @ this time; thus called a syndrome, not a disease. For those of you who have been told "but you don't look sick" and want to pull your hair out or crawl under a rock and disappear from society, PLEASE, continue reading. This book addresses all of us who have been pushed aside and labeled depressed, crazy, hypochondriacs, or lazy. FMS is a very real medical condition and this book will help empower you with information (http://www.fmcpaware.org/aboutfibromyalgia.html).

More and more data, studies, and immense progress have been made in the past few years that prove FMS is a legitimate condition. Back in 2007, the United States Food and Drug Administration began recognizing that FMS was indeed a real medical condition when it approved a press release announcing that Lyrica was the first medication approved to treat FMS. http://www.fda.gov/newsevents/newsroom/pressAnnouncements/2007/ucm108936.htm

Of EXTREME importance, The World Health Organization has given FMS its own diagnostic medical code which is accepted within the medical community across the United States. *This means VICTORY because it establishes FMS as a real and legitimate illness* making it more difficult for doctors to deny its existence, allowing insurance companies to pay your doctor for treatment of FMS, to help those who are applying for disability, and enable more research studies to be done because they can be tracked according to this assigned code. (http://www.icd10data.com/ICD10CM/Codes/M00-M99/M70-M79/M79-/M79.7)  (http://www.disabilityhelpgroup.com/fibromyalgia-finally-recognized-with-icd-10-cm-diagnosis-code/).

"As of October 1, 2015, fibromyalgia finally has its own official diagnostic code in the ICD-10-CM codes formally adopted in the U.S. ICD-10-CM, which stands for International Classification of Diseases, 10th Revision, Clinical Modification, is a list of diagnostic codes provided by the Centers for Medicare and Medicaid Services and the National Center for Health Statistics to be used for medical reporting in the U.S. The ICD-10-CM is based on the ICD-10, the statistical classification of disease published by the World Health Organization. ICD codes are used by everyone in the healthcare industry, including doctors, insurance companies and government agencies. They are used to identify and classify diagnosed diseases and conditions." http://www.prohealth.com/fibromyalgia/library/showArticle.cfm?libid=21510GB1=EM102815FGB3=EM102815FGutm_source=EM102815FGutm_medium=emGutm_campaign=FMGe=dreamweavers2%40embarqmail.com

Additionally, all of the following governmental institutions have given a seal of approval and labeled FMS a very real medical condition: The Centers for Medicare and Medicaid Services, The National Center for Health Statistics, The United States Food and Drug Administration, The Social Security Administration, The World Health Organization (WHO), and in 2012 The Social Security Administration actually made a ruling that FMS was an authentic medical diagnosis. This is pretty good ammunition!

Walk with me if you will on a journey, as a registered nurse of 22 years and also a FMS patient, down a path that will help you understand the secret and life shattering faces of fibromyalgia that only YOU can feel yet nobody can see. Our excursion will provide information to help you and your loved ones with scientific proof that fibro is real, provide a medical picture including symptoms, how fibro is diagnosed, why it's so hard to diagnose, possible causes, dissect the multiple faces of fibromyalgia, help you understand and provide ways for you to interact with family, friends, and doctors, cope and survive some of the overwhelming affects that FMS can have on your body and life, common medical treatments as some homeopathic suggestions from actual patients, research, help and useful tips for those who need to apply for disability, and exciting cutting edge information. Lastly, I have included a vast amount of testimonials throughout the entire book of people who are suffering with fibromyalgia. I believe you will find their comments to be interesting, some are entertaining, and others describe the raw truth about what it means to live with this illness.

# MEDICAL PICTURE

## MINI ANATOMY AND PHYSIOLOGY LESSON

In order to have an understanding of how FMS affects the body, it's necessary to have a basic understanding of nerves, muscles, and the nervous system. Our central nervous system contains our brain and spinal cord. The brain interprets and guides our action. The brain has two parts: a brainstem which sits on top of the spinal cord, and the higher brain. The brain stem has many parts. For our purposes we will only discuss the pons and medulla, and thalamus. The medulla controls systems in our body we don't have to think about like blood pressure, heartbeat, digestion and reflexes like coughing or sneezing, and processing sensory information. (http://www.britannica.com/science/medulla-oblongata).

The Pons (also part of the brainstem) serves as a connection between upper and lower brain. It also connects the spinal cord and brain. Think of it as a post office. Information has to go through it to get to its destination. The main functions of the Pons, pertinent to FMS, are regulation of deep sleep, and processing sensations like balance. Lastly, the thalamus, located in the middle of the brain, is also responsible for processing sensory information like taste, smell, touch, hearing, and pain. (http://www.strokeeducation.info/brain/brainstem/)

The peripheral nervous system (PNS) consists of between 45-46 miles of nerves that are outside the brain and spinal cord. They communicate over 90,000 sensations to internal organs, muscles, glands, and skin. Our muscles are wired with nerves that serve as roads to carry messages through the body, spinal cord, and then up to the brain. So the PNS communicates outside messages such as heat, cold, and pain to the brain. In patients with FMS, it is alleged we have hyperactive nerves which contribute to widespread pain. **(http://www.ikonet.com/en/ visualdictionary/static/us/the_nervous_system.**

Lastly, it is vital to mention neurotransmitter substances, or chemical messengers. As mentioned above, nerves are the roads for communication, but that communication would be impossible without chemical messengers which can excite or hamper nerve cell communication. In many diseases or disorders the flow of neurotransmitters is broken-down. The perception of pain occurs in the brain and is directly affected by communication of certain neurotransmitters, or lack thereof. These same neurotransmitters are involved in the regulation of sleep, moods, as well as thinking, perceiving and understanding. **(http://www.ncbi.nlm. nih.gov/pubmed/19479906).**

## WHAT IS FIBRO? INVISIBLE SYMPTOMS

Now that it has been established that FMS is real, we can move forward with some rationale as to why the illness has been dubbed "Invisible." Fibro is a chronic pain condition meaning the pain has lasted longer than 3 months, frequently involves anxiety, diminished social contact, difficulties sleeping, and depression (Stahl, 2009). The pain comes and goes and waxes and wanes in severity. Not only does FMS cause physical pain but also mental, emotional, and spiritual distress which will be further discussed in the next chapter. FMS is accompanied by a potpourri of other symptoms discussed later in this chapter.

According To Mayo Clinic, the chief complaints among FMS patients are widespread Pain with complaints of feeling like you have the flu, FATIGUE, disrupted sleep, sleep apnea, trouble thinking, paying attention, and focusing. Fibro patients also present with trigger points of pain on their body in certain anatomical locations which is how the rheumatological association would be able to recognize they may have a patient with fibromyalgia. It hurts when light pressure is applied to certain areas of the body-identified as trigger or tender points. Trigger points are actually tight lumps that cause a shooting pain to radiate to other areas when touched. In contrast a tender point merely causes pain to the spot and surrounding area. Trigger and tender points are identified in the picture below. **(https://showard76.wordpress.com/2011/12/02/living-with-fibromyalgia-a-guest-post-by-hayley/)**

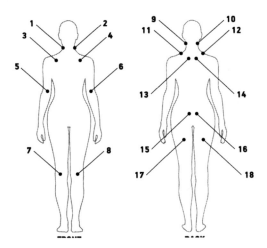

*Copyright (c) Sharon Howard https://showard76.wordpress.com/*

As you may or may not know there, is so much information on the internet and in articles that claim what FMS is, and what it is not. I am using the most reliable sources out there such as the National Institute of Health (NIH), The National Fibro and Chronic Pain Association (NfmCPA), and the Department of Health and Human Services (DHHS) as my unbiased resources to describe fibro. As you read and educate yourself I am certain you will begin to understand why healthcare personnel still want to resist the idea that Fibro exists. An understanding and some education on the part of the patient, medical workers, and caregivers may help to alleviate some stress and anxiety provoked when the "F" word (fibromyalgia) is mentioned.

Just like we all have an individual fingerprint, it is believed that no two FMS patients suffer from this syndrome in the same way or intensity.

If you are lucky enough to be female, scientists estimate between 80-90% people affected with FMS are women and approximately 10 million people are afflicted (NIH.gov). Imagine seeking medical treatment for FMS having to drag yourself to the doctor's office. Your primary complaints would likely be aches and pain throughout your whole body, constant fatigue, insomnia, headaches, balance problems, morning stiffness, brain fog, and memory problems. Those are just some of the most common symptoms. Be sure and take note that every symptom listed occurs INSIDE the body and is not observable, measurable, or noticeable like a broken leg or a green oozing wound. (http:www.womenshealth.gov, http://www.fmnetnews.com/fibro-basics/symptoms).

Often times, FMS patients walk in the doctor's office looking completely normal, but feeling like they are dying inside. When seeking help, their insides are screaming in a multitude of layers from head to toe and the following observations and statements make us cringe: "But you don't look sick. All your labs and diagnostics are normal. There is no such thing as fibromyalgia. Fibromyalgia is nothing more than a garbage-can diagnosis. I am going to refer you to a psychiatrist or psychologist." FMS patients at this point want to scream and say, "That's because I am broken on the inside, not the outside". If only it were possible to turn the patient with FMS inside out, oh the pain and damage that could be seen.

## ASSOCIATED CONDITIONS

Part of the frustration of both the physician and the patient is that there are multiple complaints the patient comes in with besides the two major ones of pain and fatigue. Migraines, autoimmune disease such as RA, and obesity (due to pain and lack of mobility) were conditions linked with fibro (http://www.health.com/health/gallery/0,,20520705_8,00.html). A cited study showed 72% of patients presented with headache and irritable bowel syndrome (IBS), 58% had anxiety, 57% restless leg syndrome (RLS), 54% depression and problems with their jaws, 50%

had chemical sensitivities, 38% had an irritable bladder, 32% had pelvic pain, and 12% had vulvodynia, or pain in the vulva, in the female patients that may cause burning and stabbing pains in the vaginal area. (http://www.empowher.com/female-sexual-dysfunction/content/vulvodynia-genital-fibromyalgia.)

## IMPACT ON QUALITY OF LIFE

Asking if FMS has a negative impact on one's life would be like asking if the pope is Catholic. It would be doing this book and all the patients suffering from FMS an injustice to not mention the impact on life. FMS symptoms range from mild to severe and vary from day to day. However, there are an ever increasing number of patients who are affected to the point of being debilitated and not being able to perform the everyday activities many take for granted. For example, getting dressed, taking a shower or bath, performing household chores, and being able to work. According to an online survey 92% of people responded that FMS had an enormous impact on major life decisions, 95% of those with children stated that it was difficult to manage their life, kids, and the household (webmd.com)

The chronic pain also interferes with and actually makes it next to impossible to plan social events. In fact, speaking for myself, I can no longer make commitments or plans because I never know how I am going to feel when I wake up from one day to the next. After multiple times of having to cancel breakfast, lunch, or shopping with friends or family, I finally just quit making plans. It's quite depressing and after a while one tends to socially isolate themselves.

In an article titled Patient Perspectives on the Impact of Fibromyalgia, I was reminded about the multiple other impacts this devastating illness has on one's life. There really is not one area of life untouched by FMS. For example, being sensitive to lights, sounds, and odors prevented participants from social events and even going to the store. Fibro patients also revealed that they believed their immune system to be weakened so they didn't want to be out among people because their susceptibility to illness and infections would increase. The other aspect that caused problems was the fact that they were physically uncomfortable in their own skin. Many described the feeling of having a sunburn. Patients also complained of other symptoms like nausea, headaches, staggering or tripping over nothing, trouble with thinking, and the lack of understanding or acceptance by others. Anxiety and psychological distress were also extremely important factors hindering quality of life for FMS patients. Last but certainly not least, the fatigue and pain that comes along with FMS in and of itself is enough to make someone want to stay home in their pajamas. (Health and Quality of Life Outcomes, Research Open Access, Disability and quality of life in patients with fibromyalgia, Jeanine A Verbunt*1,2,3, Dia HFM Pernot4 and Rob JEM Smeets3,5; Patient Perspectives on the Impact of Fibromyalgia

Lesley M. Arnold1, Leslie J. Crofford2, Philip J. Mease3, Somali Misra Burgess4, Susan C.

Palmer4, Linda Abetz5, and Susan A. Martin6

## PATIENTS SPEAK OUT

In an effort to paint a picture of what people might see if FMS was visible to the naked eye, consider the following quotes from actual patients:

-Having fibromyalgia feels like: "your body has the worst case of the flu now multiply it by 100,"

-"every nerve ending is about to explode, like someone is beating you up from the inside out,"

- *"your body is torturing you from the inside out, like having fire ants running all over your skin either biting or shocking you,"*

- *"tender and bruised in various places for no reason at all, achy, burning, stinging, throbbing pain,"*

- *"like lead in my bones weighing me down,"*

- *"like someone has a voodoo doll and you never know where they will poke or stab you, unbearable pain,"*

- *"it feels like electrical shocks in my body; my bones hurt and my muscles are sore," -"sunburned and flu at the same time,"*

- *"like you are dragging a lead ball and chain every day of your life making you so exhausted you can hardly make it through the day no matter how much rest you get,"*

*"it's every kind of pain you've ever had before roaming all over your entire body surprising you with stabs, burning, aching, bruised, sensitive to touch, and headaches". "My limbs feel like they have cinder blocks tied to them that I have to drag around; also cringing at light and sound for no reason at all,"*

*"Like I was hit all over with a baseball bat." "I always tell people that my body is just trying to implode or turn inside out again."*

There are multiple other comments from FMS patients that refer to feeling like you have been hit by a Mack truck over and over; having muscle cramps, spasms, or being hit by a car. Others say it feels like having energy sucked from your body and replaced with pain. One sufferer summed it up pretty well when writing; it feels "like someone beat the hell out of you with a baseball bat and every single muscle hurts." A last example I want to share is also a consensus among many fibro folk: on a good day you have a bad case of the flu and on a bad day you still have the flu but also it feels as though someone set your insides on fire.

## DIAGNOSIS: AN IMMENSE CHALLENGE

Because all the aforementioned symptoms cannot be seen, this contributes to the shared frustration of doctors and patients. Doctors are trained to look for causes of illness so they can treat and cure it. Patients with FMS do not provide the cookie cutter form of any illness. Unfortunately with FMS, there is no particular cause that has been identified.

For those of you with FMS, I am sure it took most of you several years and multiple doctors to get a doctor who actually took you seriously. You are not alone. A multitude of resources concur that it takes an average of three to fice YEARS to obtain a medical diagnosis of FMS. In fact, Dr. Rodger Murphree, a well-known physician and FMS guru, who wrote the book *Treating and Beating Fibromyalgia and Chronic fatigue Syndrome,* says that the average FMS patient has seen 12 doctors and waited seven years to receive an actual FMS diagnosis (Murphree 2003).

The reason is likely due to a lack of knowledge about FMS as well as it being a diagnosis of exclusion, meaning that doctors have to rule out any other underlying medical condition in order to rule in FMS. This is an extremely frustrating problem for both patients and doctors for a number of reasons. Doctors like objective, or measurable criteria. For example, a fever of 103 tells the doctor the patient has a fever, or a blood pressure of 200/120 is outside the acceptable or normal range. FMS offers mostly subjective information which means the symptoms are what the patient reports, and the doctor has to take the patient's word for it because those problems cannot likely be measured.

An additional reason FMS has been rejected is due to the fact that there is no known cause, patients don't necessarily look sick, and there are no definitive diagnostic tests or labs according to The National Fibromyalgia Association. However, the fact that there is no diagnostic lab for fibro might also be a thing of the past; more EXCITING information to come later in the book regarding this subject.

I want to make a strong statement to those of you who suffer from or think you might have from FMS. EDUCATE YOURSELF and take responsibility for your health. It is your life. As a registered nurse with my Master's Degree in Nursing with Specialization in Education who has dealt with the medical system for over 22 years, I am here to help educate and empower you, but the ultimate responsibility and power lies within you.

As stated earlier, doctors usually order a plethora of labs and diagnostic testing to rule out other medical conditions in order to rule in FMS. There are multiple other conditions that FMS could present itself as, thus it has been given the name: "The Great Imitator" meaning that FMS symptoms can mimic multiple other conditions. (www.fibromyalgia-symptoms.org/fibromyalgia_great_imitator.html.)

Unfortunately, many doctors I have consulted with fall into the category of those who do not believe FMS is real. I had a doctor look at me straight in the eye and say "Fibromyalgia does not exist. It is just a garbage can diagnosis." I was told to take control and lose weight, and then I would feel better. That statement came from a physician after I received a confirmation of FMS and education from a neurologist at Mayo Clinic just a few weeks earlier. My thought was, "Ok, really? I didn't work my way from welfare all the way up through my Master's in Nursing to decide one day that I changed my mind and don't want to work as a nurse anymore. I think not!" I was appalled and left the office in tears. It took all I had to contain myself and not explode with anger and frustration at this doctor.

# DIAGNOSTIC CRITERIA

According to The American College of Rheumatology, diagnostic criteria for fibro include widespread pain on both sides of the body, in particular tender points on the body. Initially there were 18 tender points and the patient had to have the chronic widespread pain in 11/18 of the tender points for at least three months, on both sides of the body, and above and below the waist; (http://fibromyalgia-symptoms.org/). Additionally, all other medical causes had to be eliminated.

So now that we have moved up into the 20th century, it is essential to be aware of and encouraged to know there have been multiple studies, clinical trials, and updated criteria developed to help assert the fact that FMS is indeed a real medical condition. A word of caution before proceeding: Despite the fact that way back in 1990 criteria was established by the American College of Rheumatology, according to my personal conversation with Dr. B. Gillis, 90 out of 100 doctors still want to deny the existence of FMS.

Although you may not think the following information is particularly interesting, I pray you will pay special attention to it. This evidence is going to empower you when it comes to speaking with your physicians, family and loved ones who will be resistant to admit FMS is real. In fact, you may want to go to the web site and print off the information and take it to your doctor.

In May 2010 the American College of Rheumatology proposed actual diagnostic criteria to declare FMS as a diagnosis and the system has proven to be 88% accurate. The new diagnostic tool consists of a pain measurement scale which takes into consideration the fact that FMS pain can vary in location and severity from one day to the next. This scale is called a widespread pain index scale (WPI) which does measure pain at the 18 identified "tender points." The second scale notes the symptom severity score which takes into consideration a multitude of other symptoms often present in the FMS patient. This is not a comprehensive list, but I will include the most common symptoms: Fatigue, waking up unrefreshed, irritable bowel syndrome, inability to think clearly, depression, insomnia, muscle weakness, inability to remember, and migraines or headaches. The following links will provide information for those wishing to pursue a deeper understanding of the criteria mentioned above. (http://www.prohealth.com/library/showarticle.cfm?libid=19197, http://www.fibromyalgia-symptoms.org/diagnosing-and-testing-for-fibromyalgia.html, http://www.fmcpaware.org/fm-fact-sheet)

## THEORETICAL CAUSES

Within the scope of this book, my goal is to introduce you to some theories of possible causes while not delving too deep because there is NO known cause and the information on possible causes could make up an entire book itself. I am thrilled to report, however, there has been excellent and progressive strides made and studies continue to prove there is HOPE in finding a cure and additional treatments. I do want to provide encouragement to those of you out there who are hopeless or have given up and waiting to die. DON'T GIVE UP HOPE!

There is something, however, I want to immediately mention and that is research supports that FMS is NOT a psychological condition as many physicians want to believe. Many FMS patients, including myself, are told that their illness is all in their mind. This is absolutely not true as evidenced by numerous published brain study scans. These studies support that FMS patient's process pain differently than those without it. Reference sites will be provided if you wish to see the evidence.

First let's address the more common potential causes of FMS being researched which include: bacterial or viral infections, repetitive injuries, traumatic or stressful events, patients with certain conditions such as rheumatoid arthritis, autoimmune diseases, automobile accidents, patients with a compromised immune system that have an excess of yeast (Candida) in the body, thyroid problems, vitamin deficiencies, gluten intolerances, adrenal fatigue, and bowel problems. Of particular interest to some might be the fact that there have been several genes identified that are common to fibro patients, so this could lead to genetic links. (NIH.gov).

To personalize this a bit, I'd like to share my experience with you when I had my very last trip to Mayo Clinic in regards to the explanation I received from my neurologist. I was hesitant to say the least to believe I had fibro, especially knowing there was no cure, but also knowing that I had been told so many different things by so many different doctors. The neurologist kindly took my hand and explained to me that FMS was a disorder of the central nervous system (CNS). She explained that it is a condition in which the brain does not produce enough serotonin (a neurotransmitter) which is responsible for keeping a healthy person's pain in check. Since I did not have enough serotonin, my pain went unchecked and the volume of pain was turned up loud as if turning up the sound on a radio to full blast. There was no way to control it and turn it back down. That was not my finest moment because I didn't want to believe her, but in my heart I knew what she explained was true about my pain. I have spoken with doctors since then who have told me the serotonin explanation is just a theory which has not been proven yet. All I knew for sure is that the pain was not all in my mind. It is very real.

Let's move on to a few studies that have allowed doctors and researchers to actually visualize brain abnormalities, blood flow issues, and document measurable findings between pain stimulation of fibro patients and healthy subjects. These studies open up a whole new avenue when it comes to legitimizing fibro as "real." Of particular interest is a study published online by Nichole Emerson, in the December 2013 issue of, Pain, and for the very first time ever, a relationship was demonstrated between brain structure and pain sensitivity. The exciting thing about this finding is that it could lead to better pain management. (Scans Reveal Brain Abnormalities in Fibromyalgia Patients HealthDay Nov. 3).

The next study supports the aforementioned study and was published in 2013 online in the NeuroImage: Clinical Science Digest. The study compared patients with FMS to approximately the same number of volunteer subjects who were the same age, but healthy. To state this very basically, all of the participants were placed in a Magnetic Resonance Imaging machine (MRI), had the same amount of pressure applied to eighteen of the standard tender points found in FMS patients, and afterwards they rated their pain on a scale from 0, meaning no pain, to 10, meaning worst pain in their life. One of the most basic findings showed that the FMS patients exhibited a reduced size in the medulla. Clinical correlation was made between this finding and increased pain scores when the tender points with FMS were stimulated. In conclusion, the FMS patients suffered a higher amount of pain and it was not just their imagination, it was a measurable finding. See the following web site for the actual picture of the brain scan which visibly shows tremendous evidence that the pain is REAL! http://www.lifestylehealinginstitute.com/treatments/fibromyalgia/

Neurotoxicity! This one word sums up what many functional medicine doctors, doctors who practice a combination of natural and western medicine, believe to be the underlying problem in FMS patients. To simply define neurotoxicity, it means nothing more than toxins have altered the way our nervous system communicates with itself. FMS causes sufferers to have too much NTS causing our brain to become over-electrified and a lack of the calming NTS as conveyed by Dr. Sponaugle. Serotonin, a vital neurotransmitter substance in the brain, is an important chemical that is responsible for a balanced mood, bowel function, blood clotting, social behavior, appetite, digestion, sleep, memory, and sexual desire and function, depression and anxiety, and stimulates the nausea center in the brain if something toxic is eaten. (http://www.medicalnewstoday.com/articles/232248.php).

The easiest way to describe how this phenomenon occurs is via the "Leaky-gut" syndrome. Now you may be wondering what a leaky gut has to do with the brain. I wondered the same thing myself. A leaky intestinal lining changes the delicate chemical balance of the brain. A balance between the immune, endocrine, and the nervous system starts with a healthy gut (or intestine). Let me explain: Did you know that 70% of our immune system cells "live" in our GUT!!! Plus, we have a combination of over over 500 species of good and bad bacteria in our gut which equates to 3 pounds. So imagine the bad stuff leaking into our system.

Please understand that the word "gut", medically speaking, means the intestines as well as the lining of our large and small intestines which are important for food digestion. The cells are supposed to be knit tightly to allow digested food particles to get into our blood to be used for fuel. However, many things can damage those cells that line the intestines (aspirin, alcohol, medications, stress)....AND then what happens is the cells literally get gaps in them. Think of a fish net with larger holes compared to a kitchen strainer. Obviously small things (molecules) are going to get through the fish net that aren't supposed to. RESULT: INFLAMMATION. Our immune system goes to WAR with our own body because it sees those molecules of undigested foods , toxins, bacteria, YEAST, and other wastes as fother wastes that leak into our blood as foreign enemies. Guess what? Our body is now fighting itself—sound like anything we are familiar with? This is the definition of an autoimmune disease (http://scdlifestyle.com/2010/03/the-scd-diet-and-leaky-gut-syndrome/)

So now our body starts a full blown attack which can lead to the sudden onset of new allergies. Addtionally, the leaky gut leads to nutritional deficiencies like lack of vitamin D and magnesium, like we fibro folks have. According to Dr Josh Axe if you have any of the the following nine signs and symptoms, chances are you have a leaky gut which is thought to be a major cause of many diseases and affect 80-90% of people and the results are toxic build up and inflammation:

1. **Food allergies** or food sensitivities

2. **Autoimmune disorders**, fibromyalgia, chronic fatigue syndrome or lupus

3. **Poor digestion,** bloating, gas, constipation, loose stools, heartburn and nutrient malabsorption

4. **Inflammatory Bowel Disease** (IBD), including, IBS Crohn's or colitis

5. **Thyroid issues** such as hypothyroidism, Hashimotos thyroiditis or Graves disease

6. **Adrenal fatigue, candida,** and slow metabolism

7. **Mood disorders**, including anxiety, depression and autism

8. **Chronic pain in joints and muscles,** including arthritis and headaches

9. **Skin problems**, including eczema, psoriasis, rosacea, acne and age spots

Dr. Axe is a certified doctor of natural medicine and clinical nutritionist with a passion to help people get healthy by using food as medicine. When I saw these pictures, it was like a light bulb went on in my brain and really helped me understand the association of how a leaky gut affects the entire body and causes our body to attack itself, otherwise known as an autoimmune process. With his permission, I'd like to share some photos of what leaky gut syndrome looks like, how it affects the whole body, and the association of autoimmune diseases.

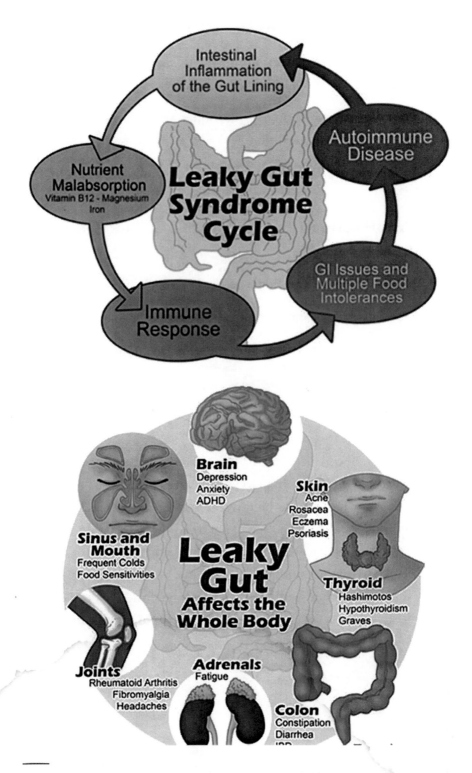

# Tissues of The Body Affected By Autoimmune Attack

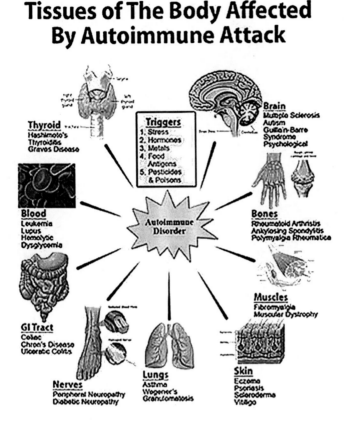

It's vital for you to realize that the yeast, bacteria, and other toxins actually migrate and deposit themselves in the coziest, fattiest organ of the body- your brain. Chemical changes then occur that affect the body's immune system and neurologic system to function the way it is supposed to. Suggestions to deal with the leaky-gut syndrome will be discussed in a later chapter. Thanks to the research of Dr. Sponaugle, who also practices functional medicine and specializes in many other medical issues, it is actually possible to see what a neurotoxic brain looks like. Courtesy of Dr. Sponaugle, this specific picture shows what a neurotoxic brain looks like, compared to a healthy brain. Clearly, there is a dramatic difference which helps explain many of our cognitive issues. This picture can be found in color at the following web site: **http:// sponauglewellness.com/fibromyalgia/**

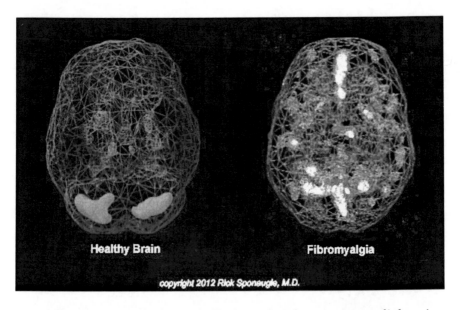

Healthy Brain  Fibromyalgia

copyright 2012 Rick Sponaugle, M.D.

I'd like to take the opportunity to share that there is some enlightening information at Dr. Sponagule's web site: **http://sponauglewellness.com/dr-sponaugle/**. He deals with many medical issues such as chronic fatigue, brain injuries, addiction, mold toxicity, dementia, and Alzheimer's disease among others. I have also visited his wellness blog found at **http://sponauglewellness.com/wellness-blog/**, which includes a wide variety of info including patient testimonies, publications, video interviews, and many other helpful pieces of information.

Moving on, there are many articles being published about FMS being a CNS disorder, which in turn is responsible for the patient's body actually amplifying or turning up the volume of the perceived pain. Dr. Clauw who is a professor of anesthesiology at the University of Michigan presented the aforementioned findings to the American Pain Society. He also added that it is believed that FMS does not allow the brain to properly process pain and other sensory information. Additionally, he outwardly acknowledges this is a painful condition **(healthheal.info)**.

Using an imaging device, single photon emission computed tomography or SPECT, a French doctor, Dr. Eric Guedj, set out to try and prove abnormal blood flow to the brain as a potential cause for FMS. The study provided some valuable information about blood flow to two different areas of the brain: 1.) The area that is responsible for interpreting the intensity of pain had too much blood flow, 2.) There was found to be an insufficient amount of blood circulation to the area of the brain responsible for emotional response to pain, and 3.) the more severe the fibro patient's symptoms, the blood circulation was immensely increased.

Dr. Eric Guedj stated this was a win-win for patients with FMS because the brain perfusion abnormalities in FMS patient compared with healthy subjects provides *measurable* symptoms thus allowing FMS to be categorized from a syndrome to a disease. He is also hoping that his findings can help doctors better understand how to help treat fibro. **(http://paintreatments.co.uk/fibromyalgia-can-no-longer-be-called-the-invisible-syndrome/)**

To further support the above study, Dr. Patrick Wood, senior medical adviser for the National Fibromyalgia Association, believed the new study provides "further evidence of an objective difference between patients with fibromyalgia and those who don't have the disorder" **(http://consumer.healthday.com)**. Dr. Wood reviewed the results but he wasn't directly involved in the research. The findings were published in the November 2008 issue of The Journal of Nuclear Medicine.

Here is some additional evidence that will help put many of you at ease and explain why you cannot process information or think clearly at times. In a math study conducted between subjects with and without fibro, researchers wanted to see the blood flow in action. Our brain has two halves, a right and left hemisphere. Solving math problems are associated with the left side of the brain. Researchers hypothesized that FMS patients would complete the task at a slower pace, because of their pain, than those without FMS. All the subjects' responses were measured for timeliness and accuracy as well as having the rate of blood flow in both halves of the brain. Of significant importance, it should be noted the **accuracy** of the responses showed no difference. However, the blood flow to the brain in the fibro patients showed something strange. Their blood flow was diverted away from the area required to solve the problem and went to a different part of the brain not associated with the task at hand.

So the brain literally re-routed its blood flow to handle what it needed to process the FMS patient's pain thus diverting blood away from the area needed to solve the math problem. This makes sense as to why patients with chronic pain complete task at a slower pace, respond slower, and are not as quick to think on their feet compared to someone not suffering from chronic pain. (**http://countingmyspoons.com/2014/11/ fibromyalgia-and-abnormal-cerebral-bloodflow/**)

When speaking of possible causes, there are multiple other theories being pursued and investigated. At the end of this chapter is a section titled "research" for those interested in reading more about what is currently being investigated as causes. The findings appear promising in way that may help control pain, find an underlying cause, or manage other associated symptoms.

## ADDITIONAL RESEARCH/RESOURCES

In conclusion, I want to remind you that there are multiple theories for the cause of fibromyalgia, none of which have been proven beyond a shadow of a doubt. However, there are many ongoing studies and research being conducted at this time. If you are interested you might qualify as a candidate to participate. I have provided web sites below for your reference if you are interested in continuing your quest on fibro.

1. Breakthrough In Fibromyalgia Research: Pain Is In Your Skin, Not In Your Head

http://www.medicaldaily.com/breakthrough-fibromyalgia-research-pain-your-skin-not-your-head-246925

2. Fibromyalgia: 5 Underlying Causes

http://drwillcole.com/fibromyalgia-5-underlying-causes/

3. Fibromyalgia and the brain: New clues reveal how pain and therapies are processed

American College of Rheumatology (ACR). "Fibromyalgia and the brain: New clues reveal how pain and therapies are processed." ScienceDaily. ScienceDaily, 11 November 2012. (www.sciencedaily.com/releases/2012/11/121111153426.htm).

4. Is Fibro Real by Gina Shaw

http://dallasneurological.com/Handouts/isfibromyalgiareal.pdf

5. Multiple Studies, One Conclusion: Some Fibromyalgia Patients Show Peripheral Nerve Pathologies

http://www.painresearchforum.org/news/33529-multiple-studies-one-conclusion-some-fibromyalgia-patients-show-peripheral-nerve

by Stephani Sutherland on 6 Nov 2013

6. Arthritis Research & Therapy : Noninvasive Optical Characterization of Muscle Blood Flow, Oxygenation, and Metabolism in Women With Fibromyalgia

Yu Shang; Katelyn Gurley; Brock Symons; Douglas Long; Ratchakrit Srikuea; Leslie J Crofford; Charlotte A Peterson; Guoqiang Yu Arthritis Res Ther. 2012;14(6).

7. Expanded list of Fibromyalgia symptoms: http://abarnabas.tripod.com/indexfibrosymptoms.html

8. Small Intestinal Bacterial Overgrowth & How It Relates To Fibromyalgia http://www.fibrodaze.com/small-intestinal-bacterial-overgrowth/

9. 100 symptoms of Fibro: http://www.fms-help.com/signs.htm

## ADDITONAL CHAPTER REFERENCES RESEARCH

Structural alterations in brainstem of fibromyalgia syndrome patient's correlate with sensitivity to mechanical pressure

Nicholas Fallon a, Jamaan Alghamdi b, Yee Chiu c, Vanessa Slumingd, Turo Nurmikkoe,f, Andrej Stancak a

NeuroImage: Clinical 3 (2013) 163–170

a. Department of Experimental Psychology, Institute of Psychology, Health, and Society, University of Liverpool, Liverpool, UK

b. Physics Department, Faculty of Science, King Abdulaziz University at Jeddah, Saudi Arabia

c. Wirral University Teaching Hospital NHS Foundation Trust, Wirral, UK

d. Department of Molecular and Cellular Physiology, Institute of Translational Medicine, University of Liverpool, UK

e. Pain Research Institute, Institute of Ageing and Chronic Disease, University of Liverpool, Liverpool, UK

f. The Walton Centre NHS Foundation Trust, Liverpool, UK

Cerebral blood flow dynamics during pain processing in patients with fibromyalgia syndrome.

Psychosom Med. 2012 Oct;74(8):802-9. doi: 10.1097/PSY.0b013 e3182676d08. Epub 2012 Sep 24.

Duschek S[1], Mannhart T, Winkelmann A, Merzoug K, Werner NS, Schuepbach D, Montoya P.

## AUTHOR INFORMATION

[1]Department of Applied Psychology, UMIT University for Health Sciences, Medical Informatics and Technology, Austria. duschek@lmu.de

Cerebral blood flow dynamics during pain processing investigated by functional transcranial Doppler sonography.

Duschek S[1], Hellmann N, Merzoug K, Reyes del Paso GA, Werner NS.

Home > October 2012 - Volume 74 - Issue 8 > Cerebral Blood Flow Dynamics During Pain Processing in Patie...

< Previous Abstract | Next Abstract >

Psychosomatic Medicine:

October 2012 - Volume 74 - Issue 8 - p 802–809

doi: 10.1097/PSY.0b013e3182676d08

Special Series on Neuroscience in Health and Disease

# CHAPTER 2

## THE FACES OF FIBRO

*Adversity and Perseverance can shape you. They can
give you a value and a self-esteem that is priceless*

*~Scott Hamilton*

Now that some groundwork has been laid and evidence has been presented that FMS is **REAL**, we can move on. This chapter moves into some pretty deep information. We will go from one extreme to the next because that is what living with a chronic illness and pain is like. Furthermore, we will deal with an up and down variety of common physical, emotional, and mental experiences; spiritual aspects, and lastly patient testimonials about the good, the bad, and the ugly. Let's start with the multiple faces of fibro.

### FACE #1: PHYSICAL

It is crucial that everyone remembers fibromyalgia is not a 'one size fits all' illness. Fibro patients are like a fingerprint, unique to the individual. In fact, Dr. Rodger Murphree, who has been dealing with

FMS patients for approximately two decades, says that no two cases of fibro are exactly alike (personal conversation, December 10, 2015).

I want to remind family and loved ones to understand that most of the pain is on the inside of the body; not able to be seen by the naked eye. However, if you really take time to look, the misery is written all over their face. Many of us try to put on a brave face, but in all actuality we wish that you could understand this statement: If you could see the pain I feel, the intensity would blind you.

Ironically, once upon a time I doubted fibro was real, and now I have been cursed with it. Living with chronic pain is like riding a roller coaster; up and down. Sometimes it hurts all over, and sometimes just certain body parts hurt. Sometimes the pain is bearable enough to function, other times you are flat on your back. The pain of fibro travels and attacks its victim minute by minute, hour by hour, or day by day. We never know when, what type of pain, or what might cause it to strike. Many will testify the pain keeps them in bed, crying, and begging for pain relief only to be told by many doctors the pain is all in your head.

According to the Fibromyalgia Network, the top ten physical symptoms of fibromyalgia include: "pain all over, fatigue, sleep difficulties, brain fog, morning stiffness, muscle knots, cramping, weakness, digestive disorders, headaches/migraines, balance problems, and itchy/burning skin." The two most common characteristics in a study published by the NIH were pain and achiness so bad that you have to sometimes hang on the wall to walk. I can attest to that. Skin sensitivity and burning were also mentioned as common painful feelings.

Did you know that there are actually seven types of pain a fibro patient can experience? Types of pain include: 1.) Hyperalgesia, which is the medical term that defines when our brain increases a painful response 2.) Allodynia is a painful response to something that would normally not bother anyone. It can cause pain to your skin just from the pressure from clothing because it feels like you have a bad sunburn. Fortunately this form of pain is rare, 3.) Paresthesia; many people associate this with numbness and tingling but it can include burning, and also include the feeling like something is crawling on your skin. Every now and then I get the sensation that I have bugs crawling up my legs. It is horrifying and keeps me up at night. 4.) Randomly roving pain: I couldn't have said it better when I found something that said my fibro travels more than I do. Pain comes and goes whenever and wherever it pleases. 5.) Sparkler burns: this is explained as tiny pin pricks of pain, 6.) Rattled nerves which includes the combination of nauseated, dizzy, and aching all over. 7.) Knife in the voodoo doll is the last type of fibro pain and means exactly what it says. It's a stabbing knifelike pain and can travel throughout your body. It can come without warning just as the rest of all these types of pain. (http:// chronicfatigue.about.com/od/whatisfibromyalgia/a/fibromyalgiapain.htm).

Fatigue is the second most common symptom of fibro. In addition to feeling like you have the flu almost every day and any other additional afflictions, imagine suffering from a punishing fatigue. Doctors say that in order to understand the fatigue experienced by fibro patients; imagine not sleeping for three days and then trying to function. In a study published by the National Institute of Health called "Patient Perspectives on the Impact of Fibromyalgia" (Arnold, Crofferd, Mease et al, 2008, October), fatigue was said to be one of the worst symptoms because it is unrelenting and interfered with every aspect of their lives.

I want to stop here and distinguish the difference between chronic fatigue syndrome (CFS) and fibromyalgia. Depending on what resource you use, there could be different answers. The arthritis foundation says that some doctors feel it is the same condition, others say it's related, and still yet, others say they are not related at all. The main differences distinguishing the two conditions are that fibro has pain as its first characteristic and fatigue second, while chronic fatigue has fatigue as its main symptom.

Common symptoms shared by both conditions include: sleep disturbances, headaches, decreased memory or attention, problems with bowels, depression, anxiety, and dizziness. Criteria set forth from the Centers for Disease Control (CDC) says that to diagnose CFS that fatigue and the following symptoms must be present for six months or greater: a sore throat, enlarged or tender lymph nodes, muscle or joint pain or other signs of systemic illness. Despite the differences noted in both conditions, treatments are similar.

Other common FMS symptoms include, abdominal pain, migraines, vision changes, craving for carbs (because your cells become insulin resistant), ringing in the ears, impaired coordination, restless leg syndrome, sensitivity to noise, lights, and temperature changes.

All of these impairments with the body increase the risk of suffering from other serious and painful health conditions. Raynaud's syndrome is often associated with FMS patients. Raynaud's is a blood vessel disorder affecting mostly your fingers and toes. When out in the cold the blood vessels constrict (or get smaller), so blood cannot get through the vessels efficiently and your fingers/toes will get cold and numb. In fact, they are likely to change colors from white to blue to red. Obviously it's important to keep your hands and feet properly protected from the cold to keep from getting frostbite or you could lose your fingers or toes (NIH.gov).

Because of dizziness, pain, and muscle weakness, studies show that people with fibro are at a higher risk for falls. I just spoke with someone from a fibro support group and she said she lost her balance, fell, and laid there for between five and six hours on the floor because she was unable to get to a phone for help. This person was not elderly. She is in her 50's. It is dangerous to be on the floor for several hours. Your body starts breaking down your muscles which can lead to multiple other serious conditions.

I have also found it to be a common theme, for fibro sufferers to NOT want to use their assist devices such as canes or walkers because they feel they are too young. Many of them are. I came across someone who was 35 and was told by her doctor to use a cane. She felt bad because she was so young and wanted to know if anyone else out there was in the same boat as she was. The stigma associated with using assist devices is terrible. I had to use an amigo when I went to the store because my hips and legs hurt so much. I was embarrassed because of all the looks I initially received. However, I got over it real quick because I made a conscious decision to not let their opinions affect me. I suggest you all do the same.

Another problem affecting fibro suffers is difficulty processing sound, sights, and touch. In turn, difficulty processing leads to overstimulation or hypersensitivity to sights, sounds and touches that would not bother the average person. This is not an imaginary issue. Using a functional MRI, a study clearly shows a decreased response, instead of an expected increased response, in the portion of the brain responsible for seeing and hearing when fibro sufferers were stimulated. Source (Arthritis Rheumatol. 2014 Nov; 66(11): 3200–3209.).

Here are the words from someone who suffered from this very condition:

> I went to the grocery store today. I had to do shopping for both my Mother (who has cancer) and myself. There were so many people and I became so overwhelmed. I began to cry and ran out of the store leaving a full basket of groceries.

Sensory overload is a big problem for me. Oftentimes my husband and daughter like to goof off because everything is a joke. Much of the time that is fine with me. However, there are times that I just want to scream and tell them to be quiet. I know when I feel like that, I am being overstimulated. I quietly tell them I need to go and lay down for a while, and I send myself to my room for some peace and quiet.

Another common theme among fibro sufferers is mood swings. As described by Dr. Devin Starlanyl on her Facebook site, she names the mood swings of brain cycling in fibromyalgia "fibroflux". Patients feel helpless to control the anger, frustration, fear, depression, and self-pity that can come and go in the matter of minutes and with great intensity at that! They may cry easily or become frustrated and angry at the slightest provocation. "Be patient and understanding with yourself, these cognitive impairments and emotional overreactions are a normal part of fibromyalgia."

A very important condition to be aware of is costochondritis which affects approximately 60-70% of FMS patients. The suffix 'itis" means inflammation. This condition is an inflammation of the cartilage connecting your ribs to your chest bone. The scary part of this condition is that it can make you feel as though you are having chest pains and/or heart problems. As a registered nurse and former cardiac intensive care unit nurse, I strongly encourage anyone with fibro experiencing chest pain to get it checked out immediately. It is important that we do not sweep all our symptoms under our fibromyalgia rug. **(http://lifeguideline. info/costochondritis-in-fibromyalgia/).**

Myofascial Pain is another ailment that is believed to be a subtype condition of fibromyalgia. Fascia is a spider web like material that connects every muscle, artery, bone and vein in our body. It covers each item both independently and continuously. Any restrictions on this system causes fascia to become thick like glue causing immense pain by exerting a pressure on its structures up to 2,000 pounds per square inch. It is said that trigger points or nodules form and when touched can cause immense pain at the site and referred pain-or pain distant to the site. The condition can be treated with regular stretching; avoiding cold temperatures which could exacerbate the symptoms, physical therapy and massage therapy which will help restore muscle strength.

Weight Gain is another side effect a fibro patient usually has to deal with. There are multiple factors contributing to this issue. During my investigation of sleep I came across some interesting discoveries. In *The Fatigue and Fibromyalgia Solution* by Dr. Teitelbaum, he links the lack of sleep as contributing to weight gain. Poor sleep leads to decreased levels of leptin. Leptin is a protein that communicates with the brain in helping to control appetite and also when we have had enough to eat. If we do not have enough leptin, our hunger is unregulated; the result will be weight gain.

Furthermore, lack of sleep also leads to the decreased production of growth hormone. No, growth hormone isn't solely responsible in helping us grow. It also stimulates the production of much needed muscle which helps us burn fat.

Probably most obvious is that FMS sufferers have a lack of mobility from pain. As stated earlier, some days are spent in bed. Additionally , the medications doctors place us on contribute to weight gain. I know that with the Gabipentin I am taking I have gained 40 pounds. I have heard many other fibro patients say the same thing happened to them. Another side effect of medications is water retention. I gained 20 pounds of fluid in a 2 week time span. This interfered with my ability to breathe and I ended up in the emergency room and then admitted to the hospital. I was treated with IV diuretics and lost 20 pounds over a weeks' time period.

So not only can the side effects be medically dangerous, the weight gain is very tough to look in the mirror and see. My self-image went into the toilet. Pictured below is a picture taken in 2009, before I got ill. Then next to it, you will see my picture as it appears on my license. I almost cried when I looked at it. I don't even look like the same person. Imagine how you would feel if this was you. As friends and family, I implore you to please show your loved ones unconditional love. They are still in there, and just need your assurance that you still love them. I can't thank my husband enough for providing that reassurance to me.

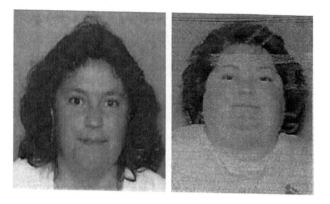

2009                    2014

## FIBRO FLARES/HOW TO COPE

As previously mentioned, fibro symptoms can come and go as well as the intensity being extreme or mild. Some days you can function to a degree and some days you feel almost well. Those are the days that are taken advantage of to catch up on household chores and running errands only to be miserable the next day and likely suffer from a flare.

A flare means that the symptoms of FMS are exacerbated and experienced more intensely. A sign of a flare could be an increase in the intensity of pain and fatigue, decreased ability to think, and even more interference with sleeping. Flares can be caused by stress, illness, injury, traveling, weather changes (big factor), anxiety, depression, particular lights, smells and sounds, overstimulation, or simply overdoing it. (http://www.fmnetnews.com/fibro-;basics/symptoms; http://www.healthcentral.com/chronic-pain/c/5949/151398/fibromyalgia/).

Obviously one way to prevent flares is to identify what your personal triggers are and try to avoid them. Also, making a list of coping mechanisms ahead of time will help prepare you. Tips for coping with flares include paying attention to triggers by perhaps journaling, pacing activities, take breaks, play mind games, drink plenty of water, medicate proactively and get the rest your body is demanding. Keep in mind that flares can last days, weeks, or even months. **(http://www.healthcentral.com/ chronic-pain/c/5949/151398/fibromyalgia/).**

Some suggestions from Mayo clinic are to pace yourself even slower than normal if you have to, provide distractions such as funny movies, word searches etc., talk to someone even if you don't want to because having support can ease your burden, and even ask for help with tasks if you need it. You may have to just say "no" if someone asks you for a favor or to do something for them. Have a positive internal dialogue inside your mind because what you think affects your perception of pain. For example, instead of saying "I can't do anything because of this illness," recite what you CAN do but tell yourself you will just have to do it at a slower pace. Other suggestions I found on a picture slide online are to get rest, drink plenty of fluids, play mind games, and medicate proactively. **(http://www.healthcentral.com/chronic-pain/c/5949/151398/fibromyalgia/).**

## TESTIMONIALS

At this time I'd like to share patient testimonials collected from a fibro support group on Facebook. The testimonies explain what it feels like to suffer with the many faces of fibro and provides a fantastic picture of the multiple faces of fibro.

The proposed question was: What is Fibromyalgia to you? Here are some of the answers provided:

> *"It is far more than pain - Pain to me is sharp stabbing etc... and I get some of that....but worse is this constant nagging ache which is worse some days more than others and NEVER gone.*
>
> *It is this fog in your thinking - like, did I turn off the stove —what did I come in here for —where did I want to go today —and those feelings are constant —the feeling that every day is dreary —overcast and cloudy even when the sun is out....the teary depression that you have no control over —you don't even know where the tears are coming from or why but you can't*

*stop them either....it is going to sleep and getting up feeling worse than when you went to bed....it is severe insomnia that can go on for days, weeks...or longer....it is having a Dr. tell you that all of your tests are NORMAL when you still feel so sick - even feverish at times....these are just a few of the things I feel EVERYDAY, ALL DAY and there are more - even as I wrap up this post I can think of some I missed but hopefully you get the drift...."*

*Fibro physically feels like "a chronic ball and chain I have to drag around every day," "It's a constant battle both physically and mentally with our bodies,"*

*"It changed me a lot very young, mine started off with attacking the muscles of my throat when I was just a teen, I began having issues swallowing. I didn't tell anyone because I was young and thought I was strange or something. It's only progressed, I became withdrawn, sad, anxious, started having my heart racing and for years I just lived afraid, afraid to eat, drink, swallow, was my heart going to beat so fast I'd die?.... . Dr.'s weren't sure what was causing the muscle and nerve problems and pain, went on for years and progressed over my whole body, I became anorexic. Just awful! ... It is a thief."*

A female fibro patient admits "frequently bumping into door frames and walls. Be careful...the stairs and door frames and flat floors that are out to get us." Sadly enough, one of the most common answers to the question was: *Fibromyalgia is a thief.* Another member admits that as she was leaving her house for work, she walked through the door way and lightly bumped her shoulder into the door jam. Next thing she knew she lost her balance and fell to the ground leaving her extremely sore. She admits her balance has been pretty bad the past couple of weeks, and she tends to trip on her own feet and pulling muscles from the falls. She tries to laugh it off, but feels very clumsy.

I would like to conclude this section with a posting originally written in the Facebook support group called Fibromyalgia Amazing Knowledge and Support (FAKS). The founder and creator of the group is Angella Phia La Ricci-Faimanifo who has built the group up to over 12,000 members and still growing.

I was so thankful when I stumbled across this site that I cried. I finally knew I was not in the boat alone. People's comments reflected exactly how I felt. It's a safe haven where I can go and share my feelings. My eyes filled with tears of joy and relief just knowing there were others out there that shared some of the same experiences I was having. It was at that point I knew I wasn't crazy.

The emotional piece of fibromyalgia is another strong aspect that prompted me to write this book. People's comments about wanting to give up, relationships and families breaking up, and the devastation it can cause to people's lives just broke my heart. I needed to to reach out and help those who were so misunderstood. One of the members, Jenna, posted a heartfelt summary that received so much feedback from others who said they could relate so closely with how she felt. I asked Jenna if I could share her posting, and she said yes. It is one of one of the most profound things I have ever read in regards to fibro.

Here is the original letter written by Jenna Ashton Roberts:

*Some people don't understand what a silent disease like Fibromyalgia actually does to a person. From the very beginning, when all of this started 1.5 years ago, this is what it has done to me. It has stolen my happiness. Ripped it right from me with no remorse. Not only has it ruined me emotionally, but physically I'm broken too. The dark circles under my eyes aren't from makeup. Fibromyalgia has taken over my life so badly, that I haven't even touched make up in over 4 months. Before this nasty disease took over my body, I enjoyed making myself presentable. I loved going out, traveling, staying up late, interacting with others, I loved getting up and going to work, I loved driving and seeing new places. The love that radiated from my body was remarkable. Now? I wake up because I don't have another choice. I have people in my life who count on me. I don't put makeup on and even if I did I wouldn't be able to cover what Fibromyalgia has done to me. I haven't wore jeans in well over 6-9 months, I can't even wear a normal bra because my body feels bruised 24/7 and the underwire hurts. I can't just hop in the car and travel last minute, I have to plan it out because being in the car is horribly uncomfortable and painful for me. I can't do anything I used to do without being accompanied by more pain than I've ever felt. My body and soul are both so tired. Tired of this disease and tired of suffering. The pain that lasts from the second I wake up until the second I fall asleep every single day, the fatigue during the day and insomnia at night, the mood changes, and the feeling of never wanting to leave my bed. That's what I am tired of. I want to be normal so badly. I want my happiness back. When I look in the mirror, I see a different person. Someone who is broken, hurt and lifeless. To everyone who doesn't understand, this right here is what Fibromyalgia does. It steals your happiness and ability to live a normal life. Each day gets so much harder. The hardest part of living with Fibromyalgia is wanting to fight back, but not having an ounce of energy to do so. I won't lie, thinking about how I will live with this disease for the rest of my life, scares me more than anything. I want to raise awareness about Fibromyalgia. To everyone out there who is living with this debilitating disease, I understand. I know what you are going through and you're not alone.*

Jenna asked me to share her e-mail address so if anyone would like to contact her, she would love to listen and help in any way possible: **Jenna.Roberts94@aol.com.**

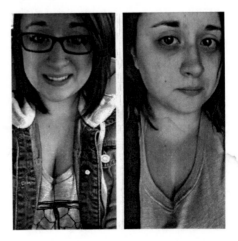

## SLEEP DEPRIVATION

I will never forget what my doctor said to me when I went into the office complaining of insomnia. His words are still seared into my brain: "if you don't sleep, you won't get well." According to the National Fibromyalgia Research Association, more than 75 percent of fibro patients suffer from a lack of deep restorative sleep which only contributes to the pain and fatigue experienced in the day. The National Fibromyalgia Association have conducted studies that confirm fibro patients awaken regularly which limits the amount of deep sleep for the fibro patient.

According to Sleep Somatics Diagnosic Center, sleep is a neurological process when the brain progresses through stages. We will focus briefly on stages three and four, because that's what fibro patients suffer from a lack of. Stages three and four are called restorative sleep and characteristics consist of no eye or muscle movement and extreme difficulty in waking someone.

The effect of a lack of restorative for anyone will have significant impacts including but not limited to memory problems, hallucinations, impaired immune system, tremors, aches, exacerbating pain, and of course a lack of energy (http://www.sleepdex.org/stages.htm). Understanding that a lack of sleep greatly affects the body's immune system, perhaps now it makes sense as to why fibromyalgia patients are at risk of developing so many other medical conditions including fibro flares.

Inability to sleep means people often need totake daily naps or rest to conserve energy just to have the ability to take care of their own personal needs. Taking a shower becomes a physically exhausting task. Household chores become neglected because fibro patients try to focus on more important chores like trying to prepare dinner for their family.

So for the fibro sufferers who are having difficulty sleeping, it is vital you find out just where your problem lies. A sleep study can be done to determine whether you are suffering from sleep apnea. According to the

NIH, sleep apnea is when you actually have a pause in your breathing, or it can be shallow breathing. Either way, the oxygen level in your blood will drop thereby causing your organs, most importantly your heart and brain, suffer from oxygen deprivation. As you can imagine, this condition poses threats such as heart attacks, heart failure, strokes, and cardiac arrhythmias **(NIH.gov)**. So as a nurse, I encourage you to speak with your physician about your sleeping patterns and ask if you might need a sleep study performed.

## HELP FOR INSOMNIA

As I was researching some sleep strategies many tips I came across were exactly as my doctor had suggested to me in order to strengthen the sleep-wake cycle (or Circadian rhythm). My doctor advised me to not take any prolonged naps during the day (no longer than an hour), wake up every morning at the same exact time, try to drink sparingly after 3pm, establish a routine by going to bed at the same time every night and waking up at the same time every day. If needed, set an alarm to wake up. Other advice: make sure the room is dark, cool, and use a fan for noise distractions; avoid caffeine after 3pm, avoid drinks after 3pm if waking is due to bladder calling, and don't use the bedroom for anything except sleeping. Can't say that I have followed all of his instructions but I am trying. Additionally, there are natural supplements one can take that will enhance sleep and build serotonin levels. These supplements will be discussed in chapter five.

The combination of pain and sleep deprivation is a double-edged sword for those with FMS: sleep deprivation exacerbates pain and pain makes it more difficult to sleep. Although there is still so much yet to be learned about the relationship between fibromyalgia and insomnia, the good news is that sleep is free, does not require a doctor's order, and creates powerful healing according to Michael J Breus Ph.D. in Psychology Today.

In conclusion, the physical effects of fibro go from head to toe. There is not one area of the body unaffected. There are so many other symptoms that can accompany FMS; In fact, too many to list here. I recently came across a resource that says there are now over 200 symptoms that fall under the FMS category. If you would like to further explore those symptoms try visiting the following web sites: http://chronicfatigue.about.com/od/whatisfibromyalgia/a/fibrosymptoms.htm, https://sites.google.com/site/lynnisaacsondesign/home/health-information-to-share/fibromyalgia--200-symptoms

## REFERENCES FOR THIS SECTION

(Mayoclinic.org; http://www.fmcpaware.org/symptoms). http://www.everydayhealth.com/fibromyalgia/101/fibromyalgia-and-sleep.aspx, https://sleepfoundation.org/sleep-disorders-problems/fibromyalgia-and-sleep

(http://www.healthcentral.com/chronic-pain/c/5949/151398/fibromyalgia/ ).

https://www.psychologytoday.com/blog/sleep-newzzz/201201/sleepless-and-in-pain-link-between-fibromyalgia-and-sleep

Arthritis Rheumatol. 2014 Nov; 66(11): 3200–3209. Altered Functional Magnetic Resonance Imaging Responses to Nonpainful Sensory Stimulation in Fibromyalgia Patients

Marina López-Solá, PhD, Jesus Pujol, PhD, Tor D. Wager, PhD Alba Garcia-Fontanals, PhD, Laura Blanco-Hinojo, MSc, Susana Garcia-Blanco, MSc, Violant Poca-Dias, MD, Ben J. Harrison, PhD,Oren Contreras-Rodríguez, PhD, Jordi Monfort, MD, MSc, Ferran Garcia-Fructuoso, MD, PhD, and Joan Deus, PhD

http://www.fmcpaware.org/m-n/myofascial-pain-syndrome.

https://www.myofascialrelease.com/about/fascia-definition.aspx

http://www.spinemd.com/symptoms-conditions/myofascial-pain

## FACE #2 & 3: MENTAL & EMOTIONAL

Along with all the physical issues, it is common for a person with fibro to experience a wide variety of emotions. Emotional and mental aspects are intricately woven together therefore will be discussed together. There are multiple issues encompassed here which include: how this illness mentally and emotionally affects patients, families, and friends; examining fibro fog and tips for managing; patient testimonials for fibro fog; tips for confronting painful emotions; dealing with grief and loss; and confronting suicidal thoughts

Many comments I read reflect that of depression, rejection by family, and the inability of physicians to believe the patients pain-thus left untreated. I couldn't believe the comments I was reading. Some examples include: I have given up; I am hopeless; I have nothing left to live for; just waiting to die; thinking of taking all my pills so I won't wake up. Several women commented about how their husbands had left them and they didn't know how they were going to get by. Another woman commented that her daughter who had two children thought she was just seeking attention so she quit coming to visit thus she lost contact with her only daughter and grandchildren.

The two most common identified emotions experienced by fibromyalgia patients are depression and anxiety. Personally, I believe it to be a much higher percentage; however some research shows that up to 30% of FMS patients experience it. Anxiety and/or depression could stem from hormone imbalances, chemical (neurotransmitter) imbalances in our brain, low blood sugar, or thyroid problems. Additionally, problems with the adrenal glands, which help us deal with the stress response, will cause fatigue, depression and anxiety (**sharecare.com**).

The adrenal glands produce cortisol which is responsible for handling long term stress. However, over a long period of time, the adrenals become stressed because of prolonged pain, thus adrenal fatigue or insufficiency occurs causing our body to experience stress overload. Personally speaking, my adrenal glands have been suppressed for years, almost every day when I wake up, my insides are quivering like a bowl of jello and I feel like I want to jump out of my skin. So I am not afraid to share the fact that I need to take meds for anxiety to help me make it through the day. The cause is physiologic, not mental. **(https://www. sharecare.com/health/fibromyalgia/health-guide/manage-fibromyalgia-pain/ steps-to-better-manage-the-mental-and-emotional-side-of-fibromyalgia).**

If you are coming from a life where you were a healthy and productive member of society, fibromyalgia will likely steal or take away some of your abilities to function. This may include the inability to work, loss of your spouse, financial hardships, and inability to be the parent or spouse you want to be; this likely leads to feelings of worthlessness, hopelessness, and inadequacy.

In a study published in Patient Education and Counseling, the authors studied Patient Perspectives on the Impact of Fibromyalgia. The outcome of the study revealed an overall negative impact on the subject's physical, emotional, social, and work realm. This study reported sleep disturbances, fatigue, pain, issues with memory, a decreased ability to concentrate, anxiety and depression, a disruption in relationships with friends and family, withdrawing from society, a decreased ability to function with their normal daily activities, lack of ability to function at a desired level thus avoiding physical activity, loss of ability to participate in hobbies or social activities, and loss of job or ability to improve their occupation. (Arnold, L., Crofford, L.J., & Mease P.J. et al. October 2008)

I'll take a moment to share a sad personal experience. It's currently February 2016, I found out several weeks ago that my own mother was expressing to other people she thought I could be faking my illness just to get attention. I was enraged because this illness has stolen my career, my ability to be the kind of wife and mom I want to be, and my ability to even get out of bed sometimes. When I found out what my mother was saying I became emotionally stressed out and devastated, which only worsens fibro symptoms. I had to make the grim decision to put distance between the two of us, thus she did not spend Christmas with me or her three grandchildren and the rest of the family.

I have experienced most of the aforementioned physical and emotional feelings of loss and grief. Depression cannot even begin to explain how I felt. After working my way from welfare to a Master's Degree in nursing with a specialization in education, I had my dream job at a community college. I do think however, I let my job consume me so my immune system was stressed and I became ill with bronchitis in December of 2010. Unfortunately, I had a life threatening allergic reaction to the prescribed antibiotic. After that, my health was never the same. Unfortunately, that's when I began to acquire a multiple health problems; my conclusion was that God was punishing me for not having my priorities in order.

Initially, I was devastated and felt useless, as if I was just taking up space and nothing more than a burden to my family. My physical capabilities left me bed bound for a while, at age 43, some nights I prayed that God would let me fall asleep and never wake up. Unlike some others, however, I have an extremely supportive husband, daughter, and friends who knew there was something terribly wrong with me. It took me a while to figure out that though I was the one that was ill, my whole family was affected. My husband carries the entire burden. He works full time, he cooks dinner almost always, does the laundry, and he and our daughter clean the house, with the exception of a cleaning lady who came in once or twice a month.

My dear daughter, Katie, who is now 12, has lived with me and my illness for six years and has adjusted emotionally to my limitations. She said to me just the other day, "Mommy, it's ok that you can't do the things with me you used to do. We will just find new things to do together." In addition, she also said, "Mommy, you know how you said you feel bad that you can't do things with me that you want to do? Well, I just have to tell you that I think you being sick has made me a more compassionate person, and well, I'm not glad you are sick, but I sure am glad you are home every day for me when I get off the bus." This mommy had tears of joy in her eyes and in heart. She is wise beyond her years.

I could go on and on and on with examples of emotional hurt this illness has caused me. Instead I decided to turn my devastation into something constructive and try to help others. Thus, here I am writing this book.

## FIBRO FOG

When I first heard this term I thought it was just made up. In fact, I even laughed out loud. Unfortunately, now I live every day with it. Fibro fog is a term used to describe all of the following: the compromised ability to think, memory loss, expressing yourself, concentrating, learning new information, holding conversations with people, trouble finding the right words when communicating, remembering where you put something, and mental confusion (http://www.fibromyalgia-symptoms. org/fibromyalgia_fibrofog1.html).

As a nurse with a Master's Degree, I cannot tell you how frustrating it is to try and carry on a conversation and not be able to speak in a complete sentence or have to ask people to repeat what they just said because your brain did not process the information. It's extremely frustrating and embarrassing. I have actually gone into my bedroom and cried at times because I felt so stupid. One of the things I used to do best, as I was told by others, was to communicate effectively and persuasively; another loss to fibromyalgia.

Causes of fibro fog are thought to be related to lack of sleep, pain, depression, and a decreased blood flow to the brain which may inhibit the creation of it new memories. Resources assure us that the condition is temporary and that there is no real brain degeneration as in

Alzheimer's. However, over time the fog can get worse. Remember it's simply problems with memory recall, not true memory loss. "Though better sleep has many benefits, some studies show there are simply different things happening in the brains of people with fibromyalgia. In one study, brain scans showed that from time to time, people with fibromyalgia do not receive enough oxygen in different parts of their brain. One possible reason is that part of their nervous system is off-kilter, causing changes in the brain's blood vessels." Mental brain fatigue and other avenues are currently being researched to help understand fibro fog. So keep your brain busy with thinking activities. (http://pain. com/archives/2011/09/30-impaired-memory-concentration/, (http://www. arthritis.org/about-arthritis/types/fibromyalgia/articles/fibro-fog.php.). http:// www.fmnetnews.com/free-articles/enews-alert-samples/fibro-fog)

## TESTIMONIALS

We have reached a fork in the road where I'd like to change the tempo to a more upbeat note. Now that we know what fibro fog is, we are going down a path that might surprise you or even make you laugh. You may be wondering how any of this could be fun or entertaining. Well, many FMS patients have learned to actually laugh at themselves instead of cry when it comes to fibro fog. I have collected quite a few examples of fibro fog that I believe you will find entertaining, and the people who shared them with me were able to laugh about it as well.

*My first embarrassing fibro fog moment: I was in a takeout restaurant alone. I needed to pee so bad, but the condition I was in at the moment (terrified confusion) I didn't want to move any more than necessary. But it was taking so long, I finally just took off towards the bathrooms. Went in, did my business. Came out of the stall & yup that's a urinal...and a man standing in front of it...I did not get my take out that day.*

*I went in a public bathroom and after washing my hands I put* them under the hand dryer, I waited and waited for it to come on, only to discover it wasn't automatic blower just a crank handle on side brought the paper towels to me!! You just have to laugh and go on!!

Ever go to a store while in a Fibro Fog, and look around guiltily to see if anyone knows you and you don't have the foggiest clue as to what you are doing? Attention shoppers: Brain Fog sale in isle 9.

I usually sprinkle baby powder in my underwear after my shower. I was sprinkling away when I noticed it was the wrong color. I was sprinkling comet cleanser.

Well I just ruined three pairs of jeans and a blouse. Put bleach in my washer of colored clothes. Maybe they will be designer jeans now. Thank you fibro fog.

I have put milk in the cupboard and cereal in the refrigerator

I find things in the fridge that really shouldn't be there.

I have so much Fibro Fog that I've lost my debit card twice in two months!!! Thankfully nothing was charged on it. I'm thinking it's probably in my purse. Lol. Got new one and lady at my bank is starting to look at me funny now.

Fibro fog? Here is my latest. I have been having a problem with these nasty little ant invasion. I emptied my cabinets and sprayed a tin of vinegar to get rid of them. I do not want to use bug spray because I have cats and do not want them to get sick. Well I have battled these little buggers for several days now. I kill them and more come in, so last night I decided to spray some bug spray because I was tired of fighting them. So I reached in my closet grabbed the can and started to spray. It looked odd. I was spraying white rustoleum paint. What a mess!

I grabbed the bottle of super glue instead of eye drops yesterday. Thank God I looked at it before putting it in my eye.

## MANAGING FIBRO FOG

Yes, fibro fog can be funny when looking at it in hindsight; however at the time it is occurring, it may not be so funny. Research suggests some of the following ways to help: get enough sleep, eat healthy, speak with and review your medications with your doctor to see if that could be a contributing factor, de-stress, do not multi-task, use a planner, and get in a routine. **(http://www.everydayhealth.com/fibromyalgia/11-ways-to-beat-fibro-fog.aspx).**

Another great idea not only from my personal experience, but also taken from research, is to write in a journal. It helps to vent and quite honestly, when you are done writing you feel a little lighter and better. According to New Life Outlook, a journal can also help you monitor your moods, look at the documentation, and perhaps identify triggers for fibro flares. I have found journaling to be very therapeutic because when I write down how I feel the paper can't talk back to me and say, "Oh if you would just get on the treadmill and lose weight you'd be fine." You can also set small goals for yourself on a daily basis. One day your goal might be to simply get out of bed, while on another day you might want to get a few things done around the house. I write my goals down on a piece of paper because when I complete a task I can cross it off. This gives me a sense of accomplishment instead of a feeling that I am not contributing to my home and family needs.

As my fibro journey continues, I continue to pick up more coping mechanisms along the way. For example, did you know that they actually make adult coloring books? While in the FAKS support group, I found out from others that you can get them almost anywhere. I recently ordered a couple through Amazon.com along with some gel pens. They are actually therapeutic coloring books made especially for adults. I've tried it and it does help. Others have mentioned they paint, and there are some really beautiful pictures shared within our Facebook fibro support group. People are proud and also feel a sense of accomplishment when done.

Another coping mechanism that has proved to become one of my "gifts," is taking pictures. I live on 12 acres and the birds and wildlife are amazing. I started out taking pictures for fun and distraction. However, as I have posted these pictures online I have been told that they look professional. I have been asked if I am a professional photographer, which made me laugh. I have received multiple suggestions that I should publish my pictures in a book or even have them used on the front of greeting cards. I guess that could be my next project after completing this book. Something that started out as a fun hobby has turned into something much bigger. You never know what twists and turns this life will bring you. Never sell yourself short.

Other ways I deal with fibro fog is to have a calendar and write everything on it including my doctor's appointments, when my injections are due, my daughter's school events, etc. I use colorful sticky notes for my to-do lists. I write myself notes and place them on my refrigerator. One funny thing with writing things down is that I do not always remember where I put the notes. Therefore I suggest placing them in plain sight. In addition to all that, I am sure to make quiet time in the morning to spend with the Lord as well as pray a lot throughout the day asking for guidance and strength.

Other sources suggest avoiding caffeine because it's a stimulant and may interfere with a good night's sleep, when you feel like you're getting foggy, take a rest break. Avoid overstimulation because, as already discussed, fibro patients can be bothered by lights and sounds. Additionally, plan ahead. Develop a plan as to what you will do when you feel lost or confused that way you have a reliable plan to fall back on and won't get so frustrated (http://www.cfidsselfhelp.org/library/lifting-fog-treating-cognitive-problems).

One more coping mechanism I'd like to mention that has worked incredibly well for me is to think positively and *focus on what you CAN do* as opposed to what you cannot do. You are what you think. For the first few years I was totally miserable and thought almost exclusively about everything I had lost and felt like nothing more than a former shell of myself. I was in and out the hospital for a multitude of illnesses and tried to stay positive and keep my faith. I tried to always have Joyce Meyer (a female evangelist), John Hagee, or Joel Olsteen on my television. So fast forward to today and I will tell you that if it was not for my faith, I would not be here. I prayed to go to sleep and not wake up on more than one occasion. I often thought about all the medications I had in my cupboard that I could help make that happen with. Thankfully, my faith gave me the hope of something better waiting for me. I knew I was supposed to still be here because technically I should have died about four times.

## CONFRONTING PAINFUL EMOTIONS

A practical piece of advice: admit that you have fibromyalgia. Psychologically, that was tough for me. I was at Mayo clinic and told by my neurologist that I had fibro. I did not believe I had fibro because I didn't want to have fibromyalgia. Denial has done nothing for me except add stress and thereby increase my pain, because stress increases FMS pain. It wasn't until just the past year or two that I finally accepted and admitted "I have fibromyalgia and it is incurable, but manageable."

As I sit and read the brochure sent to me by Mayo Clinic, it is reiterated that in order handle what is going on in your life, you must confront and be proactive. It's essential to try and stay as positive as possible and learn all you can about what you are facing. Knowledge is power (Fibromyalgia: Symptoms, Diagnosis & Treatment Brochure). Tell yourself it's natural and OK to have the feelings you do, just don't camp out there. Prolonged discouragement and anxiety lead to periods of depression, possibly isolation and thoughts of suicide.

# LOSS/GRIEF/DEPRESSION/ISOLATION

"Your life as you know it is over. It will never be the same." I will never forget those words of the Fibro counselor at Mayo clinic that caused me to sob uncontrollably: What does that mean, were my first thoughts. Is my life over? Then she proceeded with information about diet, exercise, managing stress, and a bunch of other things I don't really remember. I felt dazed, confused, and not at all ready to deal with what I was being told. My first reaction: shock, disbelief, and denial.

Living with chronic illness and pain changes people and changes life as they know it. Grieving and mourning are likely a part of daily life because guilt and pain are with us wherever we go. Not only have we lost many of our physical capabilities to an illness, many of us also lose part of our identity and long to be the person we once were. As if that was not bad enough, we often lose friends because of not being able to have any type of social life. Additionally, many often lose contact with family members because of disbelief and judgement.

The best way I know to explain the feelings associated with pain every day of your life is to share the words straight from the people suffering. Testimonies include multiple sources of loss, frustration, isolation, and anger.

> "I can't work anymore; got fired for being sick. Actually 22 months ago I applied for disability waiting on an answer. I stay in bed the majority of the time. I've isolated myself to my room."
>
> My husband has had to move to another state for work and I am alone. This illness takes more than just your activity away.
>
> Soo frustrating!! Every day I'm tired and hurt. Every day my husband looks at me in disgust. Why are you tired? You don't do anything. You have no reason to be tired. I hate it. I hate being made to feel like a worthless piece of crap. My everything hurts. Especially my heart these days.

*My husband doesn't want or care to read about it. He won't go to the doc with me either. I wish he went once or would read something so he knew something about it. Instead of complaining about I always get sick or have tons of meds, (that I don't take unless I have to) he has no idea. No one does.*

*Fibromyalgia feels like your life as you knew it just ended.*

*Fibromyalgia feels like you're being punished, mentally and physically, for even the small things you do in life.*

*I don't know what to do. My husband called me a retard because of fibromyalgia. What do I do? Where do I go?*

*I am ANGRY at people who are supposed to love me. I am tired of explaining that I don't feel good and I probably never will again. I have asked them to read about the disease....I wish they could see there are so many more people JUST LIKE ME.*

*I finished loading my stuff in my mom's car and then I get in and she tells me she is done helping me with everything, that I am dead to her. That if I was to die tomorrow she would be happy because I wouldn't be there to cause problems for her or anyone else.*

*My husband said to me last night that he thinks we should go our separate ways...*

*Tired of feeling this way. Tired of myself. I don't ask anything from anyone because I don't want to be annoying. I keep everything to myself and just go on like everything is normal again.*

After reading the comments above I think it's more than appropriate to discuss grief which commonly occurs with loss. "Grief is the process that allows us to let go of that which was and be ready for that which is to come." (http://www.drchristinahibbert.com/dealing-with-grief/5-stages-of-grief/)

As I was reviewing the five stages of grief, I came across a grieving process unique to fibromyalgia that I have never seen before. They are very similar to the original five stages of grief identified by Elizabeth Kubler Ross. Included in the stages of Fibro grief are: 1.) Denial/fear/isolation, 2.) Anger, 3.) Bargaining, 4.) Depression, and 5.) Acceptance/Re-evaluation. Although they are presented in that order, remember that the feelings may not always occur in that order, and not everyone experiences each and every stage. This is simply a guide to help us better understand common emotions many people experience with loss. Remember it is important to give yourself permission to feel and experience your feelings, but don't get stuck in a rut with any one particular stage (http://www.fmcpaware.org/ diagnosis-articles/fibromyalgia-after-the-diagnosis.html). I will take a moment to discuss each stage so everyone has a better understanding.

Denial is the first stage, which makes sense. When receiving the diagnosis, many people do not want to accept it because maybe the doctor is wrong. They want a second opinion perhaps, or they might be thinking that this type of thing happens to other people, not me. Many times fibro is a term people are not familiar with, thus they don't even know what it means; instilling a sense of fear. On the other hand, some people might actually be relieved to finally get a diagnosis.

Denial can be a healthy stage for the simple fact that it protects us from a collection of emotions that could attack us all at once causing one to be overwhelmed. Denial is a self-protective mode we go into because nothing in life makes sense, life as we know it is gone, and many wonder if and why we should go on. Denial gives us time to digest, tell our story to friends or loved ones again and again and hopefully move towards a healing process. The best thing we can do at this point is educate ourselves. (http://www. drchristinahibbert.com/dealing-with-grief/5-stages-of-grief/).

Anger is the next stage. Anger knows no limits and can manifest itself towards people for not understanding what you are experiencing, doctors for not finding out what was wrong with you sooner, or God. I was mad at the world and God. I asked the question "why" so many times. Acknowledge and feel the anger because suppressing it will only lead to feelings of guilt. Guilt often leads people to blame themselves and think they should have done something different. Give yourself permission to be angry. It is ok. Calling it what it is helps put us on a path to healing. Anger is actually an anchor of strength giving temporary shelter and structure where there once was nothing. Acknowledging anger gives way to feelings of underlying pain (http://grief.com/the-five-stages-of-grief/). It is essential to remember that anger will only elevate your stress and pain level and perhaps cause you to isolate from those you need for support. The best way for a fibro patient to deal with this stage is to mentally find the individual treatment that works best for them (http://www.fmcpaware.org/diagnosis-articles/fibromyalgia-after-the-diagnosis.html).

Bargaining means trying to find a way to get life back to the way it used to be. Bargaining often takes our mind into the past so we don't have to face our emotions or reality. It also considers many "what if" or "if only" scenarios. Many times people will try to bargain with God by promising to do anything in return for healing. Others may even find they negotiate with pain. A milestone is this stage is to keep reminding yourself that you have done nothing wrong to deserve fibro and that is not a punishment ( http://grief.com/the-five-stages-of-grief/).

Depression means you are accepting the reality of your situation. It's a normal part of the process you are going through. It involves a deep grief and intense sadness often leading to a withdrawal from the world. After facing the fact that life is a journey not a destination, I have come to realize that intermittent depression will likely be a permanent part of my life.

Life involves many stages, phases, and seasons. Each season brings different types of losses or things, I cannot do. For example, I used to be a Girl Scout leader for my daughter's troop. This illness forced me to give up that privilege. Now she is older and her interests have grown into acting in the local cast and crew who put on plays for the community. I was unable to be a parent volunteer because of my illness. I found myself withdrawing to my room and crying so many times because I am missing out on her life. My older daughter, who is married, is talking about having children soon. This would make me a grandma. I know my physical limitations are going to prevent me from being able to participate in their lives like I would want to. It's a never-ending cycle that makes you feel empty, like a burden, and hopeless at times. It makes you tired on top of the fatigue already being experienced. It also begs the question, what's the sense in going on? I haven't told many people this, but during the past five years there have been many times I would pray at night and ask the Lord to not let me wake up in the world but in heaven. I am not ashamed to admit this if it will help anyone else realize that you are not alone in how you feel. One thing that has helped me get through is coming to realize that with Fibro there are good days, and there are bad days.

Getting stuck in the hole of hopelessness could lead to long term depression. I know as a nurse and patient, long term depression can cause a change in the brain's chemistry and people might start to have suicidal thoughts. At this point, it important to recognize you are stuck and need help from a professional. You are likely going to need an antidepressant. It does not mean you will need it forever. Please understand this does not mean you are crazy. It means you are human. Again, I disclose to all of you and am not ashamed to say, I take antidepressants. One thing I caution you with, and something I experienced with antidepressants, they may make you feel more depressed and even suicidal if you weren't before. Notify your doctor immediately so they can change your medicine if you notice this happening to you.

Remember, depression is the door to the acceptance/re-evaluation phase. It's important that this not be misunderstood with thinking we are cured or that we finally fully accept the loss of our health and everything is okay. It simply means that we have reached an understanding in our own mind of what our new reality is; we have an incurable illness, and have to make the most of and move on with life. It's here where you finally realize "You can accept your pain without pain becoming your identity" (http://www.fmcpaware.org/diagnosis-articles/fibromyalgia-after-the-diagnosis.html).

In an effort to expand upon some resources to help fight this beast, I found some web sites with some great info. There is a Natural Health Advisory Institute web site with an article published called "5 Natural Depression Therapies" and can be found at the following web site: http://www.naturalhealthadvisory.com/downloads/how-to-treat-depression-without-medication-5-natural-depression-therapies-that-treat-serotonin-deficiency-symptoms-and-other-common-causes-of-depression/

I recently saw a couple postings in a fibromyalgia Facebook support group that said: "Learning to say 'NO' without explaining yourself and setting boundaries is key to developing your self-esteem. " Another posting said: "Accept what is, let go of what was, and have faith in what will be." At this point in time the realization has hit that we must spend our time and energy on our passions and purpose in life as well as what we consider to be most important. Life is too short spending it focused on negativity.

This is the stage that has enabled me to realize that my life is not over and that my purpose in life has now changed. It's why I am sitting here writing this book. Part of my energy is dedicated to finding new coping skills, thus my new hobby of taking pictures of the wildlife in my yard. Yes, the direction of my life has changed course. It doesn't have to be all bad. Much of it is the attitude we take. Life is full of surprises. I might have fibromyalgia, but it doesn't have me.

## THE BEAST

Many of us with fibro have days when we are bogged down with sadness and grief wishing and wondering if our lives will ever be the same. I know deep inside me, I hold out hope that one day I can be almost like my "old self" again. If not careful, we get easily sucked into a daily battle with extreme sadness. Before you know it the sadness becomes a slippery slope with a big pit waiting at the bottom of it to swallow you up. Inside the pit is an enemy and a beast waiting to devour you: its name is depression.

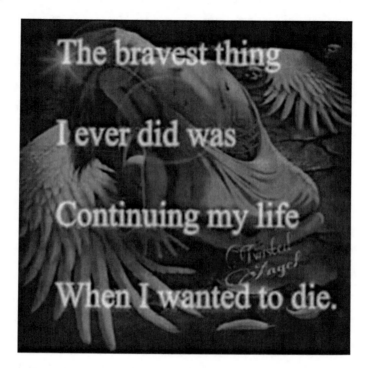

I am sure it is no surprise to those suffering from fibromyalgia and chronic pain, that research suggests we are at a higher risk for suicide. In fact, I have read that the biggest cause of death for those suffering wirh fibro, is suicide. Some research studies suggest the strong link is depression that increases the risk. We have covered a bit about depression within the grieving section. However, I want to bring into light the signs and symptoms and different aspects within this section. New Life Outlook quotes that as high as 90% of fibromyalgia patients suffer with depression. Now that statistic is more believable. The National Fibromyalgia Association defines depression "not an emotional weakness or something that you can just will away, but rather a complicated medical condition that is caused by chemical imbalances in the brain."

Signs and symptoms of depression can be emotional and/or physical and include extreme sadness, withdrawal, low energy levels, gastrointestinal problems, major change in weight (gain or loss), excessive sleep, headaches, guilt, loss of hope and worth, irritability, loss of interest in life, difficulty concentrating, insecurity and anxiety that won't go away. Additional warning signs might include joking about suicide, statements about wanting to be reunited with a loved one who has passed away, statements like I am useless, a burden, and people would be better off without me, being preoccupied with death, sudden visits or calling people as if saying good-byes, giving away personal possessions, sudden happiness, a sudden calmness, putting one's affairs in order, self-destructive or high risk behaviors. (http://fibromyalgia. newlifeoutlook.com/identifying-depressive-symptoms-in-people-with-fibromyalg ia/?keywords=fibromyalgia+depression&sessionid=nv9bdso9va4jkm3ahekh60oh a5&seealso=1)

Just to establish how seriously this illness affects people, I'd like to mention discoveries I found while researching about suicide and fibro. In an article written by Lisa Lorden Myers, she writes: "On August 15, 1996, Dr. Jack Kevorkian reportedly assisted in the suicide of Judith Curren, 42, of Pembroke, Massachusetts. She suffered from chronic fatigue syndrome (CFS) and fibromyalgia (FM). Jan Murphy, another FM sufferer, also turned to Kevorkian for help; ABCNews.com later reported her assisted suicide in the summer of 1997." In this same article she mentions a woman, age 58 from the United Kingdom, who had CFS and could not get medical help so she hung herself outside her home.

(http://www.cfidsselfhelp.org/library/killing-me-softly-fmcfs-suicide)

Suicide is a permanent solution to a temporary problem and usually occurs at the height of depression symptoms. Taken from an anonymous source, this is what depression is said to feel like:

## Q: What is depression like?

A: It's like you are screaming as loud as you can, and no one can hear. No one cares. It's like you are dying on the inside and it's slowly seeping out to your outsides. You are always alone and loney, no matter how many people are around you. No one can help and it actually hurts to smile.

Believe it or not, there are many resources to help those of you thinking of taking this route. The best advice taken from those who have attempted suicide is that if you are feeling like taking your life, talk to someone. Go to, or have someone take you to the emergency room. Call a suicide hotline number. There is a national suicide prevention hotline available 24/7. The number for the United States is 1 (800) 273-8255. The web site is: www.suicidepreventionlifeline.org.

Another suggestion came from someone who is a suicide survivor. They told me about a book called *Boundaries: When to Say Yes, How to Say No to Take Control of Your Life* by Dr. Henry Cloud and Dr. John Townsend. There's also a workbook if you desire. I looked up the price and it costs $9.57 on Amazon.com.

Lastly, I'd like to take the opportunity to share a few experiences as well as advice from those who have actually tried and survived suicide attempts. Other testimonies include people who have known someone who've tried and succeeded. I posed the following two questions to the fibro support group I am in and received the responses below: 1.) What would you say, or how would you advise someone who you suspect is contemplating suicide? 2.) If someone confided in you that they were thinking about suicide-how would you respond?

*As someone who has been there, the best thing someone said to me was that they loved me and wanted me here. Just knowing that I wasn't alone, and that someone cared enough to tell me kept me here. I have severe depressive episodes at times, and have pulled through because of others reminding me how* much I am loved. I have worked in the mental health field so I could be the person to help someone else hold on. I just had to pay it forward.

I would do what my friend did for me. He called my mom and told her I needed to go to the ER. He saved my life. I still struggle with suicidal thoughts. I have the suicide hotline number saved to my contacts.

I've been in this situation myself. My friend took me to get help to talk to someone. She used a crisis line and they were at my door within minutes. Plus she wouldn't leave my side. And I'll never be able to thank her from the bottom of my heart. My marriage was over and he tossed me away like trash after 20 yrs. BUT that didn't mean my life was over by any means, not by a long shot. So if you know of anyone who is in this position ...go to them and take them to get help ..or call a crisis line . But don't let them put you off because if the words are spoken the intent is there . And sometimes they say nothing ..so if you notice a change in their behavior ..depression for example keep a close eye on them . And lastly sometimes sadly there are no signs at all. Had a cousin who showed no signs to me thank god she's still here thanks to a sibling. Suicide is such a very complex and difficult subject to talk about. But it needs to be so more people can get the help they need.

There was a time when I was on different medicines that made me feel weird but thank God I snapped out of it! Thank God doctors changed my medicines.

I've known someone who committed suicide. Well, a couple people. So I would tell you that you would mess up people who knew you, you left a lot of garbage that has to be dealt with. You're being very unfair to the people who knew you. It's a chicken way out. You might hurt but the pain you leave any person who knew is beyond words.

*When I was younger, I attempted suicide. I was always told to go to the ER if I felt unsafe. I had two visits to the ER when I was suicidal and it saved my life.*

*I have sat with a few people that have contemplated it. You have to validate their pain and what they are going through. Then always let them know if they can wait one more day things always seem better the next day. Certainly I pray with and for them. Also offer to get help with meds if needed.*

*I've actually often thought it would be better just to end the pain myself. However not only would I not cause my daughter pain to end my own, I also have seen statistics where when a family member has committed suicide other family members are at increased risk of doing so. This is what I would tell people.*

*I would say hang on one more day. There will be a better day soon. It will stop your pain maybe but will hurt so many people.*

*Personally no one listened until I was unconscious. Woke up with them pouring charcoal down my throat in the ER. So I would mostly listen and let them know they're not alone and there's hope on the other side. You just have to hold on n don't quit. Then I would do whatever it takes to find them the help they need.*

*Immediate empathy.*

*I too fight this beast. Have for over 30 years.*

*I think my approach would be try & make them angry. I have found anger seems to mitigate the deep sorrow and feelings of the impossibility of continuing.*

*Each every time I have been asked what would have stopped me the same answer arose nonjudgmental empathy.*

*I would tell them I've been there, too, and am glad I didn't do it. I would tell them that they're in a very dark place and have lost all hope, but I can promise them that if they just hang in there, give it more time, they will be glad they did. If I had given up and given in, I wouldn't be here for my son's upcoming wedding, for example. We tell ourselves no one will miss us or they're better off w/out me, but it's not true!!! I would also see it as that person is really at the end of their rope and they need help, so I would not leave it alone - I'd be on the phone to either a family member, friend, doctor, something/somebody to get them help. Life can be really hard, bad and overwhelming at times, but I am so thankful I didn't go through with the thoughts I was having. I had to change my focus, my thoughts, my mind - our mind is a battlefield and I pray and read Scripture and it really got me through and now I'm so thankful I'm still here. I'm not who I used to be, but that's ok. I can still find things to be happy about. I would hope the same for the ones contemplating suicide.*

*Never be afraid to talk to someone, even if it is calling a hotline. Feeling this way IS NOT a weakness, we all feel down at times, and to hold things in is the worst thing we can do. I am pretty much an open book, too open at times maybe, but for the most part, it has served me well.*

This poem touched my heart and is used with permission by the author Sharon Kane from the FAKS Facebook support group:

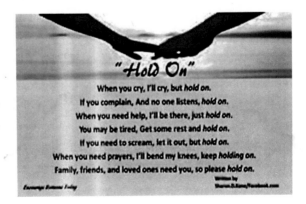

"Hold On"

When you cry, I'll cry, but hold on.
If you complain, And no one listens, hold on.
When you need help, I'll be there, just hold on.
You may be tired, Get some rest and hold on.
If you need to scream, let it out, but hold on.
When you need prayers, I'll bend my knees, keep holding on.
Family, friends, and loved ones need you, so please hold on.

## ADDITIONAL RESOURCES

Suicide Awareness Voices of Education (SAVE): www.save.org

Befrienders International: www.befrienders.org

American Association of Suicidology: www.suicidology.org

Suicide: Read This First: www.metanoia.org/suicide

National Hopeline Network: www.hopeline.com

1-800-SUICIDE

## FACE #4 SPIRITUAL EFFECTS

Not many people know what I am about to share. I am convicted to share this with you because I think it will help many people. Upon being transported to the hospital after my anaphylactic shock mentioned earlier, my husband had left that evening to tell our daughter that mommy was in the hospital. It was late in the evening and I was alone-or so I thought. I closed my eyes; I was exhausted. All of a sudden I sensed a very warm feeling at the end of a long hallway which was illuminated beyond what I can explain. Bright white light was all I could see at the end; however, I could sense the presence of people. My grandfather, whom I loved dearly and had passed away 20+ years ago, was down in the light. I could not see him, but I could sense he was there and his arms were open wide waiting for me. There was one other specific presence I could sense and it was a dear lady from church whom I had adopted as a second mother. She had died many years ago as well. There were others waiting and I started walking towards the beautiful warmth and brightest light I had ever seen. Oh, how I wanted to be there and the light seemed to be drawing me towards it. I went willingly. However, all of a sudden I felt the warmth of two hands cupping my face. Then I heard the words, "It's not your time." I immediately opened my eyes and was a little scared to turn around because I thought I was in the room alone, but then doubted myself. I slowly turned my head around to check and see if there was a nurse there or perhaps my husband had slipped back in, but there was nobody. I still felt the warmth of two hands gently cupping but not touching my face. I wasn't afraid because I knew I was in the presence of something much bigger than me.

In conclusion, I know the reason I did not give up through these past six years of hell. I know it was not my time to die. I have been given a purpose and assignment. I know now why I had to suffer with the multiple illnesses. God bless my friend Ann who so eloquently stated "Oh honey, I am so sorry you have had to endure all this agony and pain, but God is going to use all this to help hundreds and thousands of people with this book you are writing.."

Before I go any further, I want to acknowledge that spirituality does not always pertain to religion and God. In fact, the definition of spirituality can mean multiple things like finding the meaning of life, connecting with something bigger than you, someone with a priority to love yourself and others. It can also mean searching for the meaning of life. (http://www.innerbonding.com/show-article/1280/what-does-it-mean-to-be-a-spiritual-person.html, http://www.christianpost.com/news/lee-strobel-why-does-god-allow-pain-suffering-71201/)

I am not pushing religion onto anyone, in fact quite the opposite. I really don't like religion because it's not the answer. In fact it's a problem and biggest roadblock to what we should be seeking, a relationship. Religion includes man-made rules and works of the flesh. "Religion uses guilt and fear to incite works to appease which when applied results in pride." (http://definingthenarrative.com/god-hates-religion/).

Do you know that Jesus hates religion? Many people believe religion came from him. Wrong! Here is biblical proof. If you look in the bible at Matthew 23, it talks about how the high priests sat upon their thrones to make sure everyone saw that they were spiritual and to be recognized.

Religion seeks glory for man instead of God. Jesus called them fools and hypocrites. There are many other verses that also support the fact that Jesus hates religion. However, I want to get to my point I am trying to convey.

Toss out religion. Faith is all about a relationship with the Lord. The way to do this is to put all of your trust and faith in Jesus, and then accept His gift of salvation which then gives us eternal life with Him. John 3:16 tells us that "For God so loved the world that He gave His only begotten son, that whosoever believes in Him, shall not perish, but have everlasting life." It is only then that you will experience the joy of having a right RELATIONSHIP of love with God.

When going through trials, illness, or suffering many people may ask the question: So, if God is good then why do I have to suffer and endure such pain? Why didn't God create a world where we don't have to suffer? The answer is: He did. Genesis 1:31 says God saw all that He had made and it was very good. God is not the creator of evil, pain, and suffering. God created a perfect world. It was Adam and Eve that brought sin into this world through the fallen angel: Lucifer. However, Genesis 50:20 reminds us "As for you, you meant evil against me, but God meant it for good in order to bring about this present result, to preserve many people alive."

"When God reached the decision to create humankind He wanted humans to experience the greatest value in the universe, which is love. Lee Stroebel, a well known American Christian author, explains that the only way we can experience and express love is if we have the free will to love or not to love," he said. Love always involves a choice, Strobel explained. "We human beings have abused our free will by rejecting God and by walking away from Him." The result has been evil entering the world and bringing pain and suffering by the wrong moral choices people make. The other type of evil is natural evil such as disasters, he said. "This is a sin-corrupted world, not as God created it," he said.

(http://www.christianpost.com/news/lee-strobel-why-does-god-allow-pain-suffering-71201/).

For those not believing in God, that is your choice. My agenda is not to convince you, but just to spread the word and give you food for thought. I look at it this way: If I am wrong about God then I have wasted my life. But if you are wrong then you have wasted your eternity.

Before sharing a few testimonies from Facebook, I'd like you to walk through part of my journey that has deeply affected my spirituality. In December 2010 when I almost died and my health began rolling downhill like a snowball I was extremely confused as to 'why' God was allowing all this in my life. I spent the next couple years in and out of the hospital and again, could have easily lost my life a few times. One specific close call was a few days after I had my gallbladder out, I started getting an infection in my bloodstream and my one and only kidney I have, started shutting down. I then suffered from a respiratory arrest which means I stopped breathing. When I awoke to see my room filled with people and asked what happened, the nursing aide told me she came in to take my roommate's vital signs and happened to look at me and noticed I wasn't breathing. It was at that moment I surrendered and said, "God, I am tired of fighting. I give this illness to you. I can't do this anymore." Well, years later I have come to learn, that's exactly what He was waiting for me to do.

When I got home I still had major health problems and was still struggling with my faith. It felt like an up and down hill battle. I lay in bed many days and nights suffering in pain, begging God to help me. Begging for pain relief I went through stages of anger, grief, and deep depression. Simply put, I just wanted to go to sleep and never wake up. The pain was unrelenting and I questioned what in the world I had ever done wrong to deserve to suffer the way I was suffering.

I just wanted to give up and die. There are only two reasons I did not give up: 1.) my faith told me that God had a plan to use this suffering for a bigger purpose, and 2.) the love for my family. So I began a search to answer the question, "Why do we have to suffer pain or hardships? I studied many sources and came up with several answers. The first one was extremely profound. For believers the answer is found in Romans 8:17 which says as children of God, like Jesus, we are heirs to the throne. Thus we share the same inheritance as Jesus. So if we are to share in the same glory of His inheritance in heaven, then we are also to share in His suffering. Next comes the good part which keeps me looking towards having my eyes on the prize. That the suffering here on earth is nothing compared to the glory of heaven. Now that's enough to make me want to jump for joy.

I believe it to be no coincidence that at an earlier time in my life when I was also wondering WHY my biological father abandoned me at age four, I came across a sermon I had listened to in the year 2007 by Charles Stanley. The sermon was titled, "The Purpose of Trials."

Dr. Stanley explained the primary purpose we have to suffer through trials is so the Lord can conform us to the likeness of Jesus. You may be saying to yourself, well that makes no sense. Let me share with you what I have written in the back of my bible and use as a reference every time I need it. Trials purify us by causing us to turn to the Lord because He wants us to be men and women of God. He helps us face the sin in our life to free us of the bondages He does not want us to have in our life. This fits perfectly with my struggle of forgiveness and abandonment by my father. I need forgiveness and mercy, thus I need to be able to give it. We are provided many opportunities in our life to practice getting rid of the muck of envy, greed, lust, jealousy, holding grudges, selfishness etc., you get the idea.

Reason number two, to test our faith. We often face tragedies as a test of faith. God doesn't cause bad things to happen, but sometimes allows things to happen because our faith isn't strong. Untried faith is unreliable faith. If we truly trust in God then we cannot let the circumstances in our life devastate us. We have to have a deep and abiding faith. One great example I can think of is when construction workers are building a skyscraper. The taller the building, the deeper the foundation must be. Our foundation must be strong as well. Just remember, the tougher the trial the more faith, or stronger foundation, you are building.

Lastly, the Lord allows trials to show us who He is and to allow us to discover He is there with us and will help us through the trial. Many of us learn, myself included, that when trouble, pain, or trials come knocking on our door that our faith is weaker than we realized because we try to avoid suffering. He wants us to remember that He causes all things to work together for good. We are indeed allowed trials by fire. Here are a few quotes I turn to, remembering that it take a process and time, when I need comfort and encouragement:

1. God changes caterpillars into butterflies, sand into pearls, and coal into diamonds, using time and pressure. He's working on me too! ~Rick Warren

2. Remember it's the crushed rose petal that makes the perfume. ~Pastor John Hagee

3. Crisis reveals our character, often teaching us more about ourselves than we might learn in times of peace. ~Dr. David Jeremiah

4. What if trials in the life are your mercies in disguise? There is actually a beautiful song called Mercies in Disguise" by Laura Story that I often listen to when I am feeling down. You can find it on You Tube or other music apps.

5. Pressure can turn you into dust or a diamond

6. Pain and suffering have come into your life, but remember pain, sorrow, and suffering are but the kiss of Jesus-a sign you have come so close to Him that He can kiss you. ~Mother Teresa

7. Sometimes when you wonder why you can't hear God's voice during trials, remember the teacher is always quiet during the test.

8. The tiny seed knew that in order to grow, it needed to be dropped in the dirt, covered in darkness, and struggle to reach the light.

You may be asking what all this has to do with fibromyalgia. My perception is that my health problems are a trial. Each of us have trials that are suited to what the lord is trying to teach us. Like the potter who has clay. God has to work the lumps out, such as pride, anger, self-pity, impatience) and form the clay into what He wants it to be. Each of us are unique individuals with our own talents, gifts, and special purpose. We all need discipline to show us God's will and to get us out of the mindset that we should follow our own will and path. Not following the Lord's will is like saying that you know better than God what is best for your life; when in fact, God knows the beginning from the end. However that is what I said to God for days, months, and years after I lost my position as a nursing instructor. I was mad, hurt, and angry because I had worked so hard for my Master's Degree to be able to teach. My career was going full force and I was a work-a-haulic. I admit it.

As I was laying down resting and thinking about this part of my book, I was convicted to share something with you about one of my darkest times in the past 6 years. My faith was almost nonexistent. My fibro pain was so bad that it felt like someone was trying to rip my arms and legs right out of the sockets. My whole body hurt as did my heart and soul. I lay in bed with tears streaming down my face, not understanding anything in my life anymore. As crazy as this might sound, I prayed for the Lord to let me feel His arms around me and give me a hug. Then I laughed and said, I know that's impossible Lord, but I just really need to somehow feel that you have not abandoned me.

Within the next week I had a friend and former colleague I worked with in the cardiac intensive care unit, Muriel, come visit me. She said she brought me something. It was a handmade tie blanket with the pink breast cancer ribbons. She had survived breast cancer several years prior. She told me this: I made this for you so every time you wrap it around you, it will be like I am giving you a hug. My mouth dropped. Then, I became even more amazed when she handed me a book called *Hugs for Women* by Mary Hollingsworth. I opened the book and sifted through it. Believing in no such thing as a coincidence with God, I found a saying on one of the pages: "Divine hugs often have human arms-a best friend's, a mate's, a parent's. And because they are God's personified presence, it's okay to cry in their embrace....We need Him. No one else will do." I shared my story about wanting a hug from the Lord with my friend, Muriel, and cried as she hugged me. Oswald Chambers quoted "Never make the blunder of trying to forecast the way God is going to answer your prayer." So it was not impossible after all for God to give me a hug. He answered my prayer in a way I never imagined.

I have taken time to do some major reflecting on my life during this past year. After having an enormous melt down and fight with God, He revealed many things to me. First, I was so busy that I didn't have time for Him. Secondly, I was compromising my family life because I was consumed with my job. Next, I realized that His purpose for my life had changed. This was huge and changed my whole perspective because I realized that I was pursuing my dream, and not His purpose for my life. For many years I felt as though my life had no purpose, I cried so many tears I think I could have filled the ocean, I lay in bed asking God to not let me wake up, I felt like a burden, and like I was just existing. Sound familiar? I bet it does.

Now we get to the good part. I have come to realize that in order for God to use me to serve the purpose He intended I had to become *thankful* for my trials. If you are being tested, you're being perfected which means you have a divine purpose to rejoice (James 1:1-5). All this suffering I have gone through has become clear to me. The fog has lifted and I realize through the many avenues that my purpose for becoming ill has allowed multiple blessings in my life.

The first blessing is that this illness has ultimately made me know that it has a divine purpose which is to help other people with fibro. I sit here amazed that I am writing a book. You cannot imagine the doors that have opened for me to be able to do this. I have always wanted to write a book. I just had to decide what the subject would be. Well, though the door to my teaching position was closed, the Lord opened multiple other doors. For example, I always made excuses in the past not to begin writing because I didn't have a clue where to start, how to get in touch with someone who would publish it, and convinced myself that nobody would read what I had to say. Sitting here I laugh because I realize now that God had used my illness to give me more time to gain a closer relationship with Him. It's like breathing, I need Him every day of my life whether it's in singing my Christian songs, watching Joel Olsteen, Joyce Meyer, John Hagee, reading my scripture, doing my devotionals, or sharing scripture online with my Christian support group. People tell me I am an inspiration to them, and I am happy because that's my mission given by God: to share the gospel. In fact, it's the mission for all us believers.

Oh and let me share one addendum to my story above about my biological dad abandoning me when I was four. I was hurt, mad, and had every bad feeling about him that you can imagine. Throughout this time of being ill, I had to learn about mercy and forgiveness because those messages kept coming my way. Little did I know that I was being prepared for something HUGE that was about to happen in my life. In January of 2015, my biological dad came knocking on my door. I was stunned and shocked to say the least. We talked and my biggest question to him was: "WHY NOW? Why are you coming back into my life after 44 years?" His simple answer, "Because I found God. I want to be a part of your life, if you will have me." Well needless to say, this didn't happen overnight. I had to take time to process the conversations we had, but ultimately I had no choice as a believer but to forgive. God tells us if we want Him to forgive us, then we must forgive others. Folks, it wasn't easy to get past the hurt, but I prayed for strength. I am happy to say that our relationship continues to grow and after almost two years, I can look at him and say "I love you."

As a caveat, I want to share another blessing. When God opened the doors and showed me how to find a publishing company, I called the CEO and spoke with him. He was absolutely interested but there was a substantial fee I knew I couldn't afford. I bowed my head and said this simple prayer. "God, you know I don't have a money tree, so you are going to have to make a way where there seems to be no other." The following weekend when my step dad and biological dad, Larry, were here at my house, they were both aware of my aspiration to write a book. Larry came up behind me, placed his arm around my shoulder and said, "Start writing your book." I looked at him in shock and told him I didn't understand. He proceeded to tell me that he and my step dad were going to split the cost and pay the publisher, so I need to get writing because they both believed in me and knew my book would be a huge success. Sorry folks, but I do not believe in was mere coincidences that worked this situation out. With God there is no such thing as a coincidence. In fact, Albert Einstein quoted that "A coincidence is God's way of remaining anonymous." So as you can see, my testimony is that this illness has indeed brought me closer to God.

## SPIRITUALITY: FB TESTIMONIES

*I feel that this illness has brought me much closer to God. I spend time everyday praying and talking to Him. I am much more appreciative of things now, especially time spent with family.*

*My illness hasn't changed my position on God and religion at all. When I first started being open about being an Atheist, I often heard that "there are no atheists in fox holes" or some variation on that theme, claiming that I would turn to God when I faced hardship in my life. Then I became deathly ill with Pancreatitis, and spent 2 months in the hospital. That illness is what is assumed to have triggered my Fibromyalgia. But those who thought they knew my mind better than I did were wrong. At no time did I turn to a belief in prayer, a higher being, or an afterlife as a way to comfort myself.*

As for me personally, I know this illness has me seeking a closer relationship with Him....as I prepare myself for the day ahead I talk to Him and ask for healing and quote healing scriptures daily. I keep the faith that "by His stripes I am healed" no matter what it looks like or how I feel. The Bible tells us that we have to speak those things that be not as though they are and I believe the bible when it says the power of life and death lies within our tongues....

In summary, there is no part of our body, mind, spirit, and soul that is left untouched from the effects of fibromyalgia, chronic pain, or chronic illness. We all inevitably go through different seasons in our life that will cause us to grieve; nevertheless, we don't have to let our illness become our identity. There are multiple things we can say and do to help not only ourselves deal with the challenges, but also help the people in our lives. We can enhance our interactions by educating ourselves and loved ones to build our relationships so they become stronger. Yes, our lives and relationships will face challenges, but there are ways to cope. We can be like that tree in the wind that bends but does not break.

# CHAPTER 3

---

# THREE MAGIC WORDS

*Communication must be HOT.*
*That's Honest, Open, and Two-Way*

*~Dan Oswald*

Disbelief, judgement, and accusations that we are faking it can be worse than fibro pain itself. Again, because the illness is not seen, it has been nicknamed an invisible illness. To be honest, it made me not only nauseated and heartbroken, but also angry to hear the words "but you don't look sick..." For those of you not aware, there is a web site called **butyoudontlooksick.com** for patients with chronic illnesses. Look it up!

People with fibro do not desire sympathy. We want you to accept and believe what we are telling you. When you don't it causes feelings of abandonment and rejection which in turn causes a gap in the relationship. So what are those three magical words people in chronic pain long to hear from family, friends, and loved ones? **"I BELIEVE YOU!"**

I need to take this one step further because of the feedback I received from those who suffer from fibro and chronic pain. While it is imperative that people believe our pain, we want to know you are going to be here for us. Other needs include the following. I am quoting here: "Validation of the illness is totally required!" We need to hear the words "I am here for you." Because as someone rightfully pointed out, just because someone says they believe you, doesn't mean they are going to stand beside you.

Fear of rejection is absolutely valid. I have seen one testimony after another where a person in chronic pain has lost their loved one because they are not the person they used to be, because they can no longer "do" the things they could once do, or because their illness has prevented them from meeting their partner's needs. I ask the question here: What ever happened to the wedding vow, "In sickness and in health?"

Do you really think millions of Americans suffering from the same cluster of symptoms are faking illness so we can go through countless medical procedures, many of which are painful or uncomfortable? We have been poked, prodded, invaded, put on medications and suffered countless side effects. Many of us have lost friends, careers, and are no longer able to play with our children or do the things we once loved. Does that sound like something that someone would say they want to be when they grow up? Please understand that it's not the illness we fake, but rather we try and fake being well so we can have some type of quality of life. Needless to say, that doesn't always work, which leads to feelings of failure or being inadequate.

## WHAT YOU SHOULD KNOW

A few things to remember about chronic pain; it is exhausting. I don't believe there is a single body system that goes unaffected. It stresses our physical bodies and adrenal glands which are responsible for enabling us to deal with stress. Adrenal problems can cause heat or temperature intolerances, poor sleep, make us crabby, withdrawal from social activities, kills the ability to concentrate, can damage self-esteem, and weakens the immune system making us more susceptible to illness. That being said, keeping sick people away is a good idea. **(http://www.webmd.com/pain-management/guide/understanding-pain-management-chronic-pain).**

Chronic pain can come and go, feel less severe one day but be excruciating the next. It's not stress, it's not imaginary, it's not a figment of our imagination, we are not crazy, and it's not our fault this has happened. We stress over not being able to meet our role demands such as being a good spouse or parent. We strain over things that should be easy and it takes us longer to complete a task than it would an average person. Please understand we are in pain, not stupid.

In an article titled "8 Things to Remember If You Love Someone With Fibromyalgia" published on line at medical health news info, there are some vital points people living with fibro and chronic pain want you to know. Yes, some of the points might be redundant, but they bear repeating because over 25 million people just in America suffer from chronic pain, which is believed to be an under-reported number.

Here are eight critical points that communicate why chronic pain suffers endure more than meets the eye:

a. Chronic pain is INVISIBLE. Many times those suffering look fine because they have learned to "deal with it "for fear of drawing attention to themselves. We can look fine, yet be crying on the inside.

b. It often leads to depression because being in pain can easily lead to isolation, withdrawal, and strains relationships.

c. We often don't know how it started unlike those who suffer from an injury and can at least understand why they feel like they do. Without reason, the pain seems meaningless, bad luck, or something deserved.

d. We don't know if it will ever end. Living in a world of the unknown is frightening. So facing the fact that we will live the rest of our lives in pain, does not provide such an optimistic future most of the time.

e. We blame ourselves. We often beat ourselves up with feelings of guilt, being self-critical, feeling like a burden, and guilt ourselves into blame if we cannot fight the pain.

f. We are not making a mountain out of a molehill. Because the pain/problems cannot be viewed, it's easy to make a judgement about how the person looks on the outside. I have seen a statement that correctly communicates "If you could see the pain I feel, the intensity would blind you." No judgements please.

g. It's exhausting. Chronic pain fluctuates. Some days it takes every ounce of energy to get out of bed, some days plans might have to be cancelled, but the one thing to remember is that those of us in chronic pain need your understanding, giving us a break, and planning low energy activities.

h. We appreciate your support. Feelings of apathy, frustration, and hopelessness are not uncommon for those with chronic illness or pain. So having someone who will listen, offer support, and be non-judgmental is key. http://medicalhealthnews.info/8-things-to-remember-if-you-love-someone-with-chronic-pain/

## THE SPOON THEORY

So what is a good way of explaining to anyone just exactly what it's like to try and make it through the day suffering from chronic pain or illness? I have discovered something called the "Spoon theory."

A woman by the name of Christine Miserandino has developed a rather ingenious way to explain what daily life is like when living with a chronic illness. "The Spoon Theory" uses a spoon as a way to measure one task or unit of energy. The person living with a chronic illness has only a certain amount of energy to get through the day, and each day our energy reserves vary. So let's say on an average day we have 12 spoons, or units of energy to make it through the entire day.

When I wake up in the morning and get out of bed, take one of my spoons away because just getting out of bed is a chore. Making breakfast and taking my meds costs me another spoon. If I have to take a shower, that likely costs me two spoons. So right away I have lost four spoons and its likely only 9 or 10 am. That leaves me with only eight spoons for the rest of the day. In all actuality, we often run out of spoons before the end of our day, and having a negative amount of spoons is an absolute possibility.

For those of you interested in watching the video yourself, there is a you-tube video of Christine Miserandino explaining her "Spoon Theory." It can be found at the following web site: **https://www.youtube.com/watch?v=jn5IBsm49Rk**. I urge you to go and watch this video if you have not already. Then, have your significant other, family, and friends view it. After my husband and dad watched it you could actually see a light-bulb moment of understanding occurring. It made me feel better to know they had a much better idea of what it takes for me to get through a day. My husband and I sometimes joke about how many spoons I have left, or if I do something in particular, how many spoons it might cost me. This lightens the mood yet gives him a good understanding of how I am doing overall.

## HOW TO COPE: FAMILY RELATIONSHIPS

Prior to moving forward, I want to acknowledge the fact that I know it is not easy for a family or spouse to deal with their loved one who is chronically ill. It causes stress and strain on the relationship, possible financial hardship, and difficulty in watching a loved one suffer knowing you can't take the pain away. Many times coping skills are absent and marriages and families fall apart. This is another main reason I am writing this book. If I could help just one family from breaking apart, all my efforts will have paid off.

Many times, family and friends may not know what to say to someone in chronic pain, so they end up saying something that only makes it worse. This section is dedicated to helping fibro sufferers, family and friends gain some insight as to things they can say and do to be helpful. On the other hand, I will also mention some things you should not say or do. Please understand, everything I mention is something suggested by either myself or others suffering from a chronic illness/FMS.

Speaking from experience, I was so miserable with this illness that I did not initially realize let alone acknowledge the hardship my family was suffering. Thankfully I finally came to my senses and realized that when one part of the family unit suffers, the whole family suffers. The following paragraphs offer some practical advice I have learned along the way from myself and others dealing with fibro, chronic illness, or chronic pain that you can use to help preserve your relationship.

Often times in your relationships, loved ones feel helpless or, at the very least, like they are not doing enough to help you thus contributing to your illness. Be sure to tell them that it is not their fault and gently explain you don't have the energy or feel well enough to participate in activities you aren't up for. As fibro sufferers, we often try to hide or fake it and suffer through activities because we want to do things with the family. However, then we end up suffering ten-fold because we over-extend ourselves. Speaking to women, I want to say we often expect our spouse to instinctively know things. This is a dangerous mistake. We must take the lead and include our partner in planning within our boundaries.

Be honest. If you are in terrible pain, and need to cry, go ahead. But try not to shut your partner out. Don't be afraid to let them know exactly how you are feeling. If you shut them out then they will think you are doing ok that day.

While it is true you are in pain, so are they. Acknowledge their pain. They are suffering with you. Remember to take those small moments to provide comfort to them as well by offering the words: Thank-you for all you do, I appreciate you, I respect you, I love you. Be sure you thank your spouse for their support, love, and encouragement. As I write this, I am reminded of a quite by John Grey from the book Men are From Mars, and Women are From Venus that says "Men are motivated when they feel needed..." Remember to simply say thank you and tell them how important they are to you.

Please, ask for help from outside sources, if they are available, to reduce some of the burden on your spouse. Seek out sources like friends from church, neighbors, and family members; whatever it takes. It can be as simple as having a friend help clean the house or prepare a meal. This can certainly reduce the strain on your relationship.

Your spouse is likely feeling the weight of the world on their shoulders. I know that when my health crisis took the final turn and I had to go on disability, we lost my income as a nursing instructor. I was working at a community college making decent money. So I went from a well paying job, to a measly long term disability check. Don't get me wrong, it is better than nothing, but the burden of providing for the family fell on my husband's shoulders. The debt didn't decrease, but our income was decreased significantly. He also had to do laundry, cook, clean, and hold down the fort as I was in and out of the hospital for some pretty serious illnesses that could have easily taken my life. Add to that the every day stress life brings like getting our daughter to and from school and working full time. Looking back I often wonder how he held up.

Lastly, I'd like to address romance and sex in your relationship. It's often quite difficult for someone who is ill to convey to your partner that you are too ill, or too tired, without hurting his or her feelings. One of my favorite sayings comes to mind here: Honesty is the best policy. Many partners don't know that when someone is ill that the desire for sex is lessened. In the case of severe illness, the desire is often non-existant. Many times medication can play a part in this process by decreasing your libido. Help your partner realize that. However, you can find ways to express physical love and affection without forcing yourself to have sex. The most important thing is to openly communicate and be honest about what's going on because your partner cannot read your mind. I would like to conclude this section with a poem dedicated to our loved ones- used with written permission from the author, Ruth Levi-Kent who lives in England.

## If I could

Did you really hear me?
Did you take it in?
That Fibro is a problem
It hurts from deep within
It hurts from the outside too
Not that you can see
Most of my body is in pain
A painful poorly me!
Just to lift my arm up
Or to try to brush my hair
It's tiring and it's tender
You would see if you were there
As for getting dressed
That will take a while
To rest and recover
Then it's past lunchtime.
I used to take for granted
All the things that you can do
Now it's such an effort
To raise a smile for you
If I could go back in time again
To times when I was well
I would do it all again
And give my body hell!
I would run and jump and swim and ski
And dance the whole nightlong
Just to be like you again
What I wouldn't give
To have the life that you have
To get up get out and live...

© words and photo Ruth Levi-Kent www.facebook.com/Fibrolight

## HOW TO COPE: RELATIONSHIP WITH CHILDREN

Vibrant, alive, active as vice president of the parent teachers association, co-leader for my daughter's Girl Scout troop, field trips with the school, attending parent teacher conferences, volunteering for school parties; this was life before my illness. Now I get tired just thinking about it. It's all gone. I have had to give it all up and I sure feel guilty, worthless, and like a bad parent at times. Our children depend on us to be there and care for them; however this illness has forced my sweet daughter to help become my caregiver. When this illness began, she was only five years old and scared of losing her mommy. She was confused and didn't know what to think which made it hard for me to know what to say or do. After all, I am the parent. Aren't I supposed to know what to do or say to comfort my child? Just because I am ill doesn't negate the fact that I am still a parent. So how do we cope with illness and raising kids?

The first and most important thing is to let them know you are still there for them and you still love them. Though I experienced so much guilt when I had to step back from the activities I was involved in, I try the best I can to make it to parent teacher conferences, take an interest in what she did at school that day, ask her to see any papers she brought home, and ask her all about her day. The important thing to remember is that we cannot over extend ourselves or we will spark a flare, becoming sicker, which is not going to help you or your child. Another huge challenge I faced with my daughter was her concern that I was going to die. Once I was home and stabilized from some life threatening occurrences, I took the time to sit with her and explain that I wasn't going to die, but that it was going to change my life because I felt like I had the flu every day and that I was in pain all the time. She understood that because she knew it hurt for her to even touch me at times. It took time and understanding on both our parts.

Although every child is different, and of course based on their age, I found it important to let her help. My daughter was so proud that she could help by getting me a glass of water. It's important, however, that you let them know you are still the parent and they are not responsible for your well-being. Please know that there are age appropriate books out there, written specifically to help younger kids understand when they have a parent living in chronic pain or with a chronic illness. I found a book on Amazon.com called *How Many Marbles Do YOU Have?: Helping Children Understand The Limitations of Those With Chronic Fatigue Syndrome and Fibromyalgia*, written by Melinda Malott that uses marbles as a metaphor to help children understand mom or dad's limitations.

Lastly, and probably most important, show your children you love them. My daughter walked in one day as I was having a "moment" of guilt and tears because I couldn't do the things with her I wanted to. She was old enough to understand what I was feeling, so I explained my feelings. She gently and lovingly said to me, "Mommy, its ok that we can't do the things we used to do. We will just find new things to do together." What a bright light for me. We now share special times snuggling at night before she goes to bed watching movies, we play Yahtzee together, and we even color together in my stress relieving coloring books. She remains a happy and thriving child.

## OTHER RELATIONSHIPS

I'd like to share a heartfelt testimony from someone suffering from fibro and chronic pain. For a very long time this person felt as though she was not being heard or believed. Oftentimes it is misunderstandings and lack of communication that leads to hurt. I would venture to say that there are many family and friends out there whose response would be similar.

Please read this with an open heart:

*"This past Saturday I confronted my dad and told him how I feel about my pain. I told him I have taken every medicine, tried every diet, and seen every diet, nobody can help me. He listened to me and then broke into tears saying, "I feel helpless, you are my baby I want you to feel better; I want to take away your pain. You don't deserve this" For the first time in my life I felt like someone was listening to what I was saying.*

When it comes to maintaining friendships, don't feel obligated to explain or educate acquaintances regarding your illness. If they ask, it's another whole issue. However, it's not your responsibility and you are not a designated PR person for fibro or chronic illness. Chances are if you do engage in a conversation to explain yourself it will lead to defensiveness or misunderstandings. Both of which are not beneficial to you or your health.

For friends you have a closer relationship with, perhaps you can suggest they watch the Spoon Theory, or they can read or download the following letter: "Fibromyalgia? Because you asked.... The letter is located at the following web site: **http://www.prohealth.com/library/ showarticle.cfm?libid=18971**

To conclude this section on coping and communication with family and loved ones, I have compiled a list of suggestions of things that might be helpful to say versus things that would NOT be beneficial and would most likely be very hurtful for the patient suffering with a chronic illness.

| Worst things to say | Helpful thing to say |
|---|---|
| But you don't look sick at all | I know you look ok, but I accept you are suffering beyond what I can see |
| No one ever said life was fair | You don't deserve this |
| Everyone gets depressed at times | I love you |
| Maybe you should take some vitamins | You are brave |
| You just need a hobby | Let's pencil it in |

| | |
|---|---|
| Just pull yourself together | I care about you |
| You have no reason to feel this way | You are doing all you can |
| Snap out of it will you? | Tell me how you feel |
| It will pass | Tell me about your illness |
| You have it so good, why aren't you happy? | I miss you |
| I thought you were stronger than that | That must really hurt |
| Just try a little harder | How can I help? |
| It's all in your head | I believe you |
| Just drink more water | This is not your fault |
| There are a lot of people worse off than you are | I am not going to leave you |
| I am sorry (we don't want pity or sympathy) | I am here for you |
| You're just having a bad day | Do you want a gentle hug? |
| At least you don't have to go to work/ or school | You are important to me |
| You should try……. | I understand you can't control it |
| Maybe you just need to rest | You didn't cause this |
| Maybe if you exercise and lose a little weight…. | I'm here to listen |
| You need to get out of the house more | I understand if you need to cancel our plans |
| My other friend had that and she is fine now | I have no idea what you are going through |
| Disease is all in your mind | Do you want to talk about it? |
| God only gives us what we can handle- He picked you because you are strong | Sometimes it feels like we are given more than we can handle |
| Well at least it's not cancer | I know you must need someone to just vent to occasionally. I may not fully understand how you feel, but I'm here to listen anytime |
| It must be nice to stay home and relax all day | Do you have an errand I can run for you before coming over? |
| It will get better, just be patient | How can I help you? |
| You take too many medications | Don't feel bad if you have to cancel plans at the last minute, I understand |
| Maybe an anti-depressant will help | Are you up for company today? |

| | |
|---|---|
| You have what? I've never heard of that | I Googled your illness |
| Aren't you feeling better yet? | What do you wish people understood about your illness? |
| Are you still sick? | I want to understand |
| I wish I had time to take a nap | Can I visit, call, email or text? |
| You're just getting older | I know how hard you are trying |
| It can't be that bad | Can I bring you food? Can I come over and help out around the house? |
| Tough it out | I know how hard this was for you- thanks for using your energy to spend time with me |
| You just need to have a positive attitude | Here's a funny story |
| This too shall pass (chances are it will not) | I recognize this may likely never go away |
| Are you feeling better today? | I'd like to pray for you now if that's ok |
| When you just don't know what to say- say this: | |
| *I wish I knew what to say, but I do care about you and I'm here for you* | |

## COMMUNICATING WITH DOCTORS

I hate to break the news to you, but honesty is the best policy. There are more doctors out there who do not believe fibromyalgia is real as opposed to the ones who do believe it's real. I had a conversation with Dr. Gillis, a researcher, who stated that 90 out of every 100 doctors you come across do not believe fibro is a real condition.

Therefore, unless you have the good fortune to be under the care of a physician who is experienced with fibromyalgia, your doctor visits could be among the most stressful experiences. When we fall ill, we naturally expect doctors to help us. We expect them to be knowledgeable, caring, and considerate. When your doctor proves to be none of those things, perhaps dismisses you with a shrug, suggests you see a shrink, or implies that your symptoms are fabricated, it can be devastating. That's why I am going to provide you with crucial information in how to select the right doctor, how to prepare yourself for your doctor visit, appropriate questions to ask, and also provide you with web sites that you can print off and use as tools for additional communication with your physician.

Just like you would not go to a dermatologist for heart bypass surgery, most physicians are simply not trained in treating fibromyalgia. That doesn't make them bad doctors unless they say "I don't know what's wrong with you, so YOU are crazy." If they do that , stand up, give them a big hug, and tell them " Thank you for letting me know up front what an utter nitwit you are, so I don't waste my precious time on you." Then walk out the door. A rheumatologist is likely who you will see when it comes to diagnosing fibro and will likely offer Lyrica, Cymbalta, or Savella. However, let me off this advice. A functional medicine doctor is more familiar with this illness overall. For more information on this subject see **www.ABIHM.org** or **www.Naturopathic.org.**

Selection of the right doctor is imperative for the treatment of fibromyalgia and any other chronic pain condition. As a nurse and patient with complicated medical issues, I chose to see an internal medicine doctor as opposed to a general family practice doctor. The main difference between the two is that an internal medicine doctor completes an extended period of education, approximately three years, and treats adults with more complex cases. As with many fibro patients, I am dealing with multiple conditions that overlap and make my condition extremely complicated. So complicated that after 4 visits to Mayo Clinic, they sent me away confirming my fibro, but not knowing what else was wrong with me. They told me I was a medical mystery.

On the other hand, a family medicine doctor can provide comprehensive care including promotion of health and disease prevention which focuses on the patient-physician relationship in the context of the family. They treat children up through geriatrics. If you have a family physician you trust and one who believes in fibro, then I say stick with them.

However, there are doctors who genuinely care for their patients and suffer from feelings of intense frustration when they cannot help them. In the case of FMS, this experience is all too common. Doctors may feel guilt, helplessness, and a loss of self-confidence when their patient returns week after week, without having received any benefit – and in many cases, having gotten worse – from the treatments they have recommended. Doctors are only human, after all. And FMS is one of the greatest challenges they will face as a medical professional. Not all doctors are able to stand back and admit they are not up to it.

## BE PREPARED

Whether you are seeing a doctor for the first time or a returning patient, it's imperative you are prepared to communicate effectively. I had a physician tell me the average visit time with a patient is 8 minutes. Of course there are exceptions to that rule, especially with specialists, but the point being, you will be much more effective if you go in prepared and armed to communicate and present your case efficiently.

Keep in mind that fibro is second only to osteoarthritis as the most common rheumatologic disease. (Healthheal.info). The question remains, how do I find the right doctor? Rheumatologists seem to be the go-to doctor and are the most knowledgeable in diagnosing fibro because they follow the diagnostic criteria and standards set forth by the American Rheumatological Association.

Items to consider when looking for a doctor are as follows: a doctor who believes fibro is real, a doctor who is familiar in treating fibromyalgia, one who believes in working collaboratively as a team, one who listens to you and is empathetic. If you absolutely still have no idea where to go for a doctor, here are some suggestions I have gained from others as well as my own experience through the years. Ask a friend, preferably a nursing friend, or someone in the medical field who works around doctors. If possible, ask your family doctor for a referral to a rheumatologist, neurologist, functional medicine, or pain management doctor. Go to a local fibro support group and ask which doctors those patients are using and then go home and do some research. Lastly, you could call your health insurance company and ask for a list of doctors or even specialists who accept your insurance. At the end of this chapter I have listed a multitude of available resources to guide your search for a doctor.

## WHAT QUESTIONS TO EXPECT DURING YOUR VISIT

In chapter one, I introduced the tender spots that doctors may use as pressure points to check for pain, but I want to provide additional crucial information. They are still going to evaluate whether you are experiencing pain within the areas pointed out on the graph in chapter one. Based on the following information, if you meet the criteria, you can then be diagnosed with fibromyalgia.

Be prepared to answer the following questions as well as rank the severity of each of the problems.

1. During the past 7 days rate the following as no problem, slight problem, moderate problem, or severe problem.

   a.) Fatigue

   b.) Trouble thinking or remembering

   c.) Waking up unrefreshed

2. During the past 6 months have you had any of the following symptoms: yes or no

   a.) Headache

   b.) Depression

c.) pain or cramps in the lower abdomen

1.)    The physician will be looking for any other condition that could explain the pain- this is where the difficulty comes in having to rule out other causes of your symptoms.

(Reference **drfirooc.com**)

As a nurse and fibro sufferer, I have a knowledge base I'd like to use that I believe will help you avoid a flat-line relationship with your physician.

1.  If you have any previous unpleasant experiences with physicians believing in fibro, leave them at home. Don't walk into the office with pre-conceived notions that this visit is going to be like every other one. Doctors are trained to read body language. In fact, the words we speak are but a small percentage of how we communicate.

## WHAT MAKES AN IMPRESSION?

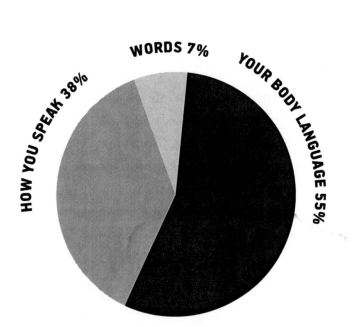

2. Communication Suggestions:

a.) Don't Whine: More times than not when we visit a doctor we are tired, frustrated, and exhausted. It's easy to get caught up in the "poor me" attitude. This will only make it easier for the doctor to dismiss your concerns or label you as a drug seeker. However, I assure that you will make much more progress if you go in with the goal of communicating your concerns constructively. Deal with the facts, not emotion. Now there have been occasions when I have had tears, and there's nothing wrong with that. This is much different than what I mean than by being whiny.

b.) Don't Lie: Many patients don't tell the complete truth about what they have tried whether it's sharing a prescription from a friend, over the counter meds, herbal meds, or whatever the case may be. Not telling the complete truth can be dangerous.

c.) Don't be defensive. Don't go in with the thought "Here we go again. Another doctor who is just going to tell me I am crazy and want to throw pills at me." Walk in with an open mind and a positive tone. It can make all the difference in the world. If it doesn't, then it's time to find another doctor.

d.) Don't look for sympathy. While it is always nice to have a doctor with a great bedside manner who shows compassion, let's face it, they are all not like that. Given the choice of a good bedside manner or a top of the line doctor, I would choose the later. I can get compassion and empathy from my friends, husband, or fibro support group. I want competent medical care.

e.) RESPECT. In the end it's about a mutual respect between doctor and patient. We need to LISTEN. There is a difference between hearing and listening. When we hear- we are usually thinking in our mind of our own response thus not really registering what the speaker is saying. We want to be listened to, and we should also listen to them. Here are some ways to show respect and listen:

## SOUNDS LIKE

*One person speaking*
*No Interruptions*
*No Solutions*
*Clarify' what speaker said*
*Wait for pauses*
*Paraphrase*
*Ask relevant questions only*

## FEELS LIKE

*Speaker is important*
*Calm*
*Understanding*
*You are paying attention*

## LOOKS LIKE

*Hands in lap*
*No fidgeting*
*Lips closed*
*Eye contact*
*Relaxed and attentive*
*Nod head*

3. **Be prepared!** It is your job to communicate in a clear, brief, organized way. Write the information down in a small notebook or on a piece of paper, so you won't have to struggle with remembering and you will. Here are some guidelines as to how you can do this. Suggestions are as follows:

a.) Where is your pain?

b.) How long you have been in pain?

c.) Rate your pain on a scale of 1-10.

d.) What makes your pain better or worse?

e.) What meds or treatments you tried?

f.) Be SPECIFIC about how your symptoms have affected your life.

g.) Be prepared to ask questions- here are just a few examples:

1.) Why do I have good and bad days?

2.) I don't understand why my pain travels through my body.

3.) How do we know if I have fibromyalgia?

h.) Make sure you write your questions down prior to your appointment.

After being a patient for 6 years and seeing nearly 50 doctors, I was tired, needless to say, of trying to remember all my symptoms. I simply couldn't because my brain couldn't process information and the fibro fog was atrocious. Therefore, I came up with an awesome tool to use Now I simply hand this chart to the doctors and tell them to keep it with my medical records. My method was simple. I started at the top of my head and went to the bottom of my feet and listed every single symptom I experienced. I also tried to include how my illness interrupted my ability to function and live my daily life. I also included things that have been stolen from my social life such as my ability to be a Girl Scout Leader, be in the PTO, and even work as a nursing instructor anymore.

I'd like to share this information with you. Please be aware, I don't mind if you model a chart like this, but make sure you plug in your own information. Make sure you are completely honest with your physician. It's imperative you don't just jump to the conclusion that you think you have fibro, when indeed it could be something else. This information is provided as a guideline only. Please note that at the end of this chapter I will be providing web-site links for pain assessment tools you can refer to and print off if you are interested.

| Head to Toe Documentation | | |
|---|---|---|
| **Symptoms** | **How long? How often?** | **How it interferes with my daily life** |
| Blurred & Double vision | 6 years/ daily | Causes headaches, unable to focus vision clearly, not safe to drive |
| Migraines | 6 years/weekly | + nausea, have to go to bed in a darkened room, incapacitates me |
| Foggy headed, forgetful/confusion | 6 years/ multiple times a day | Unable to process information, unable to think clearly, cannot safely drive |
| Dizziness | 4 years/ daily | Lose my balance and fall approx. 3-5 times a week |
| Muscle pain all over entire body | 6 years/ every single day | Unable to perform simply daily tasks, bed bound some days due to pain and weakness |
| Fatigue | 6 years/ all day every day | Unable to clean house, vacuum, meet my personal needs, need help getting dressed, need a shower chair, bed bound some days, unable to cook for my family….. |
| Inability to sleep through the night | 6 years/ 6 nights a week | Wake up unrefreshed, unable to think straight, inability to leave home, frequent naps if possible |
| Pain-generalized and in joints | 6 years/every day | Hard to walk, wake up stiff and stay that way for hours, inability to function and interact with family leads to depression |
| Unable to tolerate noise | 6 years/ 5 days week | I cannot be around a lot of people, go to the stores because I get overwhelmed, I have to go into my room and close the door |

I would also like to add the fact that I have missed every single school event in my daughter's life, cannot even attend Girl Scout events with her, and am unable to even attend church. I think I was able to go to church twice within the last six months. I am basically homebound.

I am going to stop here: I am sure you get the idea now

## EXPECTATIONS FROM YOUR DOCTOR

1. Don't expect your doctors to be miracle workers. Tell them you would like their support, but that you know your illness is quite complex. Ask for their expertise and cooperation.

2. If a doctor tells you that the illness is psychosomatic (all in your mind), or that you are simply depressed and need to exercise, **MOVE ON.** Don't try to argue with him or her. It is discouraging when doctors dismiss you, but it is a waste of your time and effort to try to change entrenched ideas, no matter how right you are.

3. Ask your general practitioner for a referral to a specialist if they are unfamiliar in dealing with fibro, more specifically a rheumatologist who does treat and deal with fibro patients.

4. If you have a trusted doctor, bring him or her educational materials. It is best to limit the materials you share with your doctor to medical research abstracts/articles or articles written specifically for physicians. Reputable doctors are not going to consider blogs written by patients or forum discussions to be credible information.

I recently had to change my rheumatologist because my previous one went out of private practice. On my second visit to her, I asked her if she had heard of the new fibromyalgia blood test that Dr. Gillis had invented. She told me no, but was intrigued. Of course, I just happened to have printed off the information and handed it to her. I then asked her if she would be willing to order the blood test for me, she agreed. She was open to learning more. I went in prepared, well informed, and had a suggestive, not demanding, demeanor. You are much more likely to get further if you communicate in that manner as opposed to walking in and telling the doctor what you read on the internet and start making demands. As a nurse of many years, I have a lot of experience communicating with physicians, please trust me on this one.

In conclusion, the bottom line is communication on both the giving and receiving end. Understand that if you are the ill one in your family that it not only affects you. The whole family as a unit is affected and most likely it will impact the way your household functions. The best thing you can do is inform and educate yourself and family to keep your family intact as opposed to letting them slowly come apart at the seams. Chronic illness affects the fabric of a family as a whole, so do all you can to continue informing and coping effectively.

## REFERENCES FOR YOUR FIBRO TOOLBOX

1. Fibromyalgia Pain Assessment Tool

   Answer 12 questions at the following web site to learn more about the pain you are experiencing. Then you can take the answers to your doctor:

   http://www.fibrocenter.com/fibromyalgia-pain-assessment

2. Having a Good Conversation With Your Doctor May Not Always Be Easy:

   http://www.fibrocenter.com/discussing-fibromyalgia

3. 10 Questions You Should Ask Your Doctor About Your Fibromyalgia:

   http://www.emaxhealth.com/8782/10-questions-you-should-ask-your-doctor-about-your-fibromyalgia

4. Preparing for your doctor appointment: by Mayo Clinic Staff:

   http://www.mayoclinic.org/diseases-conditions/fibromyalgia/basics/preparing-for-your-appointment/con-20019243

5. The American Chronic Pain Association Communication Tools: EXCELLENT SITE

   https://theacpa.org/Communication-Tools

6. Seeing a Fibromyalgia Doctor: How to Make the Most of Your Visit

   http://optimalwellnessctr.com/seeing-a-fibromyalgia-doctor-make-the-most-of-your-visit/

7. Agency for Healthcare Research and Quality: How to ask tough questions to your doctor

   Podcast: http://healthcare411.ahrq.gov/radiocastseg.aspx?id=706&type=seg

8. Agency for Healthcare Research and Quality Be Prepared for Medical Appointments

   Podcast: http://healthcare411.ahrq.gov/podcast.aspx?id=278

9. Finding the Right Fibromyalgia Doctor: What to Ask About Treatment When Choosing a Doctor:

   http://optimalwellnessctr.com/tag/choosing-a-doctor/

10. Your First Visit to a New Doctor:

    http://www.painfreelivinglife.com/daily-living/everyday-activities/your-first-visit-to-a-new-doctor/

# CHAPTER 4

---

# THE MIND BODY CONNECTION

## AM I CRAZY?

---

*You will face many defeats in your life, but never let yourself be defeated.*

~Maya Angelou

I am willing to bet that almost every person reading this book, who is ill, has either thought or asked themselves "Am I Crazy?" I confess that I have thought and asked this of myself at least 100 times if not more. The short sweet answer is: NO. These symptoms are not a figment of your imagination. If you have doctors tell you that "it's all in your head" then it's time to find a new one. There is plenty of evidence out there now thus no excuse for doctors to be uneducated about this condition. In the book The Fatigue and Fibromyalgia Solution by Dr. Teitelbaum, I laughed aloud when he called any doctor who tells you that this is all in your mind, a nitwit; more specifically an "unscientific nitwit."

I found myself quickly identifying with Dr. Teitelbaum's comments that during his 35 years of practice he realizes that most CFS/MFS have a type A personality, take care of everyone, except ourselves, and are extremely empathetic. This makes for a perfect storm and creates within us a toxic dump because we drain ourselves of energy and slowly wear ourselves down over a period of time. This is thought to be a major contributing factor for our enemy we now know as fibromyalgia.

As a fibro sufferer, I want to share information that has helped me significantly. The very first thing we all need to remember is that "everywhere you go, there you are." Don't write me off as crazy just yet. Let me explain. We all engage in "self-talk." In other words, we carry on internal conversation in our mind with ourselves. With that being said, the conversations we hold with ourselves should be as positive as possible because of the connection between the mind and body. Positive thoughts equal a positive attitude as well as an increased sense of well-being. Negative thoughts equate to negative chemical reactions, discouragement, and perhaps a loss of hope.

Prior to introducing coping mechanisms I'd like to provide medical evidence and give examples of actual studies that show the power your mind has over your body; both positive and negative. Then I will provide information to empower yourself so you don't have to drown in your circumstances. I am not saying that there won't be challenges, hard days, or rough times. I am not suggesting we bury our head in the sand and pretend our problems don't exist either. But if you take a moment and be honest with yourself and are willing to admit it; we as humans tend to automatically think the worst or jump to the most awful conclusions. Our brains are wired that way as a defense mechanism. However, I am going to deliver some very interesting facts that should help you examine your thought life and how it could be affecting your overall health.

*Rule your Mind or it will rule you*

*Horace*

The best way to describe the mind-body concept is the interaction between our body, thoughts, and the outside world (*Mind and Body Connection-Attitudes Affect Your Health by Patty Carrosicia*). The mind and body are inseparable. This has become an intriguing field of study in science called psychoneuroimmunology which says the mind and body are inseparable. Additionally, it explains thatour emotions and attitudes affect not only our health but our medical treatments and outcomes as well.

The National Institute of Health calls the connection between the mind, body, emotions, immune system, and neurological system a biochemical connection. What that simply means is that all the same hormones, chemicals, and psychological processes are used to communicate messages between all the aforementioned systems. But did you know you actually have the capability of changing the structure and function of your brain? Technically this is called neuroplasticity. In essence, you can re-wire your brain or thought processes. **(http://nmrnj. com/positive-thinking-improves-physical-emotional-health/)**

Let me differentiate the mind versus the brain. The brain is the storehouse or computer of our body. The mind consists of our mental attitudes and I liken it to the software we download into our computer **(Takingcharge.csh.umm.edu).**

I found some amazing scientific proof that thoughts can **physically** affect you in a positive or negative manner. Prior to giving you some incredible examples, I have some practical examples such as those you may have seen on the news. A young man suddenly becomes trapped under a car when the jack fails as he is changing a tire, and his father is able to lift the car enough for the young man to crawl out. Yes, that's our adrenaline coming from our fight-or-flight reaction controlled by our nervous system. There are multiple ways our emotions dictate our actions on an everyday basis and I am going to prove the interrelationship as well as the power these emotions can have over an individual.

You may have heard about this first example I am going to provide called the broken heart syndrome. This is a real phenomenon and according to **heart.org** the proper medical term for it is 'stress-induced cardiomyopathy' or Takotsubo cardiomyopathy. Physically it means part of your heart becomes enlarged and does not pump blood effectively. The good news is that if diagnosed and caught it is treatable and reversible.

As I was researching for an example to share, my heart was breaking. I came across a story about a woman age 29 who was elated when finding out she and her husband were expecting their first child. She was extremely healthy and anxious to fulfill her dream of becoming a mom. However, 12 days after her due date, she was induced into labor, only to deliver a stillborn baby. As she cradled her dead baby, it was reported that only five hours after delivery she lost consciousness and died of a broken heart because after an autopsy was performed, no other cause of death could be found. It was speculated she wanted to go be with her baby **(www.mirror.co.uk/news/real-life-stories/broken-heart-syndrome-now-doctors-1418375)**.

I am sure many of you have heard about older folks who have been married for 30, 40, 50 years and when one spouse dies, the other one seems to follow not too far behind. When there is no plausible health reason to explain the death, they diagnose it as broken heart syndrome. That leads me to the statement the mind and heart are intricately connected.

Here is a fascinating example that can be found in the book *Getting Well Again*. There were two oncologists who encouraged their patients to visualize their cancer as broken pieces of hamburger meat. Then they were told to imagine that their white blood cells, which serve as an army in our immune system, were gobbling the hamburger up. Interestingly enough, the patients who did the visualization in combination with their medical treatment lived TWICE as long as those who did not do the visualization exercise. (*Mind Body Connection, Patty Carrosicia*)

Here's something that grabbed my attention. There's a book called *The Sacred Balance* written by Davis Suzuki which speaks of how poisonous words can be. He discovered that condensed molecules that were exhaled from the breath of negative verbal expressions such as disgust, rage, and distrust contain enough toxins to kill 80 guinea pigs (http://www.collective-evolution.com/2014/04/11/the-effects-of-negative-emotions-on-our-health/).

I am going to ask you to recall back in chapter one when I spoke about neurotransmitter substances and how they relay messages throughout our body. This next example actually involved a brain scanning device which allowed researchers to measure timing of the electrical signals. Researchers in this project wanted to investigate the impact of negative words on the brain. Subjects were placed in the brain scanning device and researchers monitored the brain and what happened when the subjects were told the word "No." The results: brain signal functions were disrupted. While this temporary disruption was not harmful to the subjects, it does provide evidence that over a prolonged period of time negativity is likely to cause depression, which is defined as disruption of brain signals.

Let me provide one more example for those who might remain skeptical. As a nurse the placebo effect is intriguing to me. A placebo, or decoy drug, is basically a fake form of medical treatment. It is often used in clinical trials when studying the effectiveness of new medications. Please note: It is a law that patients have to give their informed consent to participate in drug trials and they do not know whether they are getting the actual medicine or not.

I went back into some archived information and found a study where patients were misled to believe they were infected by a dangerous bacterium and thus treated with a placebo. In reality there was no infection and the treatment was a placebo. Results were astounding. Some of the people actually developed symptoms of an infection. Their mind convinced their body they were infected with bacteria which in turn enforced their immune system to respond as though they were dealing with a harmful infection (http://www.bibliotecapleyades.net/salud/esp_salud35.htm).

Time to switch gears and look at the sunny side of emotions and the powerful effects of positive thinking. When I was in nursing school I remember writing a report and referencing an article where a man was diagnosed with incurable cancer. He was told to go home and get his affairs in order because he had less than a year to live. However, this man did not listen to the doctors but instead went to the video shop and rented funny movies. He watched funny movies for every waking moment over an extended period of time and lived a very long time. The doctors couldn't believe it when he went back because the cancer was gone and could not be found on any scans performed. There was no medical explanation for it except that laughter is the best medicine. Then again, that's not a new finding for me because Proverbs 17:22 says "A joyful heart is good medicine, But a broken spirit dries up the bones." (http://biblehub.com/proverbs/17-22.htm).

I'd like to discuss placebos in a positive way. As quoted byDr. Deepak Chopra, thinking is "real" medicine, as proven by the placebo effect. When patients were given a sugar pill instead of a prescription drug, an average of 30% of the patients showed a favorable response. Expectations are a powerful tool and if the mind-body connection causes you to think you were given a medication to help you then the power of your mind can trigger your immune system into starting to fight an infection that is not even there. How Powerful! (http://www.cnn.com/2011/12/05/health/positive-thinking-deepak-chopra/).

## CREATING A TOOLBOX

So now that you have all this mind body connection information, you need to create a tool box and formulate an action plan. I am going to discuss multiple ways of dealing with the many negative thoughts that come into your head. However, we all have our own individual personalities, likes and dislikes, and personal preferences. So please remember that every single one of the suggestions or thought processes will likely not apply to you. Pick what works best for you, or deviate and develop some of your own.

Start with ONE technique. Don't try too many things at one time because you will become overwhelmed which could cause you to give up. I will briefly remind you of some examples of people who tried and tried and failed before they were successful. Henry Ford went completely broke 5 times before he successfully started Ford Motor Company, Harland David Sanders' aka Colonel Sanders chicken recipe was rejected 1,009 times before a restaurant finally accepted it, Thomas Edison's teachers said he was stupid and he failed 1,000 times before inventing the light bulb, Orville and Wilbur Wright battled depression and failed many times prior to building the first plane that could fly, J.K. Rowling, author of the extremely successful Harry Potter series, was a single mom, broke, divorced, on welfare, and severely depressed prior to writing her novel series. You may be asking what any of this has to do with fibromyalgia. Well, the answer is simple. Many people with chronic illness and pain want to give up. I know I did. The answer is not to give up, but to get up every day with a new mindset because you are loved, worthy, beautiful, and irreplaceable. You woke up because there is a reason for you to be here on this earth. It might not be for you, but instead to be a blessing to someone else. I look back and thank God that He didn't answer my prayer to let me go to sleep and never wake up. Obviously He had a much bigger plan than I was aware of. Please remember, this journey is going to be a marathon, not a sprint.

If you don't make peace with yourself- you declare war on yourself. In simple terms, you can think yourself sick. Stress or negative thoughts affect the body, mind, emotions, and behavior and are not just unhealthy; they are destructive to your body. Negative emotions triggers the amygdala in the brain which is involved in the processing and expression of emotions, especially anger and fear, to activate our fight or flight reaction. In other words, adrenaline comes to the rescue to help our body's perceived threat. So when the body is in the fight/flight mode we are able to less defend ourselves against illness because the body's self-repair mechanisms and immune system become compromised. (mindbodygreen.com).

Additionally, chronic stress and negativity has been found to decrease one's life span. Science has discovered that negative attitudes, helplessness, and hopelessness actually damage and shorten the end caps of our DNA which play a large role in aging. So be sure not to feed into the negative thoughts like "I'll always be sick, My family all gets cancer, I am going to die young" because chances are your thoughts will lead to a shorter life span.

## PHYSICAL EFFECTS OF NEGATIVE EMOTIONS

Unfortunately those of us living in chronic pain cannot take that stress completely away, it is likely a fact that we will live in a certain degree of pain due to our illness. We may not have complete control over our physical bodies, but we surely do have a choice as to how to deal with it.

I'd like to take a moment to share with you a visual diagram. It shows the organs affected by negative emotions such as stress, worry, anger, frustration, envy, anxiety, sadness, depression, hate, impatience, and fear (just to name a few). It also shows some of the negative effects on our health. See the image on oposite side.

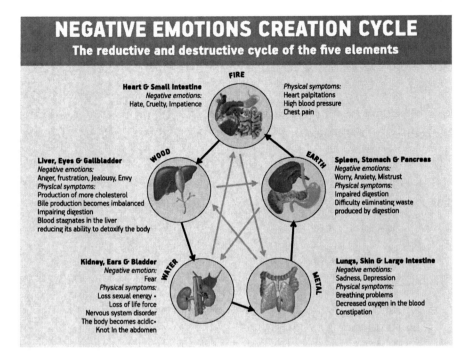

## NEGATIVE EMOTIONS CREATION CYCLE
### The reductive and destructive cycle of the five elements

**FIRE**

**Heart & Small Intestine**
*Negative emotions:*
Hate, Cruelty, Impatience

*Physical symptoms:*
Heart palpitations
High blood pressure
Chest pain

**WOOD**

**Liver, Eyes & Gallbladder**
*Negative emotions:*
Anger, frustration, Jealousy, Envy
*Physical symptoms:*
Production of more cholesterol
Bile production becomes imbalanced
Impairing digestion
Blood stagnates in the liver
reducing its ability to detoxify the body

**EARTH**

**Spleen, Stomach & Pancreas**
*Negative emotions:*
Worry, Anxiety, Mistrust
*Physical symptoms:*
Impaired digestion
Difficulty eliminating waste
produced by digestion

**WATER**

**Kidney, Ears & Bladder**
*Negative emotion:*
Fear
*Physical symptoms:*
Loss sexual energy •
Loss of life force
Nervous system disorder
The body becomes acidic•
Knot in the abdomen

**METAL**

**Lungs, Skin & Large Intestine**
*Negative emotions:*
Sadness, Depression
*Physical symptoms:*
Breathing problems
Decreased oxygen in the blood
Constipation

I'd like to provide evidence that stress actually exacerbates, or worsens the pain of fibromyalgia. The scientific study by Fischer et al shows evidence via the testing of increased stress hormones, namely cortisol which increases when the automomic (automatic) nervous system is activated. The difference in this test is that the pain is actually measurable, or objective, as opposed to relying on self-reported pain or subjective information. Prior to the study, researchers hypothesized that stress would cause an increase in pain. For 14 days women carried an I-pod to answer questions prompted to them throughout the day. Right after they answered the questions they were to collect samples of saliva on themselves in addition to collecting samples when they immediately awoke in the morning. It was no surprise to the scientists; people in pain had higher levels of measurable cortisol in their blood. There is a bit more information on this study if you wish to investigate. (http://countingmyspoons.com/2015/10/study-shows-stress-increases-pain-in-fibromyalgia/)

Let's face it, FM and chronic illness is no picnic. At one time or another we have all focused on negative influences that impact our attitude whether we realize it or not. You'd have to be a robot not to let that occur. Ask yourself this question: Are my thoughts stressing me out? I know mine were so I had to make a choice as to whether to continue to live in misery or change my thoughts. A couple ways to change your thoughts include having realistic expectations and not feeling sorry for yourself. Do not be led by your emotions because they are not dependable. As stated by Joyce Meyer, "Victory is pretty much impossible until we learn to live beyond our feelings."

According to **healthheal.info**, there are definite things we should be specifically aware of that shift our focus to an undesirable one when dealing with the prospect of living with chronic pain and illness. The first issue is the most obvious: pain. When we are in pain, let's face it, we're more likely to have a negative frame of mind. It's especially hard to be optimistic when we hurt. However, if you remember how thoughts affect our physical well-being, we need to put our best foot forward and think as positively as possible. Try focusing on just one thing in your life that makes you happy. It can be your family, grandchildren, the beautiful flowers, working in your garden, or anything. Remember- your body hears everything your mind says- stay as positive as possible.

Defense! Since fibro and chronic pain is either misunderstood or not visible to the naked eye, many times we hear the statement: "But you don't look sick." Those of us who suffer from chronic pain know what an infuriating and frustrating statement that is. We can either let our blood boil or we can chose to not feel the need to defend, justify, or validate ourselves.

Living with chronic illness provides many opportunities on a daily if not hourly basis to feel miserable. As already explained earlier in this chapter, we can add to that feeling of misery and pain. I want to provide information from an article that explains six mental thoughts and actions that can also make you feel inferior in so many ways.

1. Feeling sorry for yourself: Do not give negative feelings power over your mind. Yes, there will be times when we are sad and upset about what is going on in our life. The problem is staying stuck in that rut of negativity. It's like being stuck in the mud with your car and your wheels just keep spinning and you sink deeper and deeper into depression. Over the many years I have had a lot of practice in this area, so I spent time digging my way out of a hole. Here are some thoughts that helped me:

   a.) Helen Keller tells us that self-pity is our worst enemy and those who give way to it can never do anything good in this world.

   b.) Our feelings are visitors, let them come then let them go.

   c.) Our struggle is part of our story.

   d.) Perhaps the butterfly is proof that you can go through a great deal of darkness, yet become something beautiful.

   e.) Sometimes you will be in control of your illness and other times you'll sink into despair, and that's OK! Freak out, forgive yourself, and try again tomorrow.

   f.) Sometimes it takes an over-whelming breakdown to have an undeniable breakthrough.

2. Wasting energy on things on things you cannot control: The first thing that comes to mind with my fibro pain is that a change in weather makes my pain worse. That is when it's time to pull out your trusty toolbox and cope the best you can. We are going to talk about building a toolbox (or collection of coping mechanisms) in chapter 5. Stressing out and worrying only causes more pain. There are many things in life we cannot control, but we can control our thoughts and how we react to what occurs in our lives. Some words of wisdom that have helped me deal with this issue include:

a.) Worry is like a rocking chair. It gives you something to do, but doesn't get you anywhere. ~Joyce Meyer

b.) Why use your mind to worry, when you can use your heart to pray?

c.) Worry occupies the part of your heart where faith should live.

d.) Worrying will never change the outcome.

e.) Worrying is stupid. It's like walking around with an umbrella waiting for it to rain.

*~Wiz Khalifa*

f.) Worrying does not take away your problems or troubles, it steals your peace.

3. Trying to please everyone: Anyone with chronic illness knows this just is not possible. Whether you are a mom or dad with chronic pain or illness, you know that some days are nearly impossible to function let alone live up to the responsibilities you have. So ultimately you are going to let someone down, including yourself. This is where we have to try and not let guilt get the best of us. Here are some thought that have helped me cope:

a.) Learn to say No without explaining yourself because setting boundaries is key to developing your self-esteem.

b.) Be yourself. You are beautiful just the way God made you. You don't need to be accepted by others. You just need to accept yourself.

c.) The key to failure is trying to please everyone.

d.) The sooner you stop trying to please everyone, the sooner you will be happier.

*~Chumzee*

4. Expecting Immediate Results: I know I am guilty of expecting results to occur overnight sometimes. However, change takes time.

When making positive changes in our life, say for instance dietary changes as I am now, we cannot expect to see all our weight melt off overnight, in a week, or even in a month. This illness has caused me to gain lots of weight, so I have to be patient and positive while I wait. My goal every day is to not give up. I have to renew my mind daily and accept the truth of reality in my heart and mind. At this moment in time, I am working on lifestyle changes which include dietary and activity level changes. I am seeing progress which encourages me to keep going. So focus on the positive gains, even if they are baby steps. Here is some encouragement:

a.) Happiness is a journey, not a destination.

b.) You can find inspiration in everything, if you can't look again. ~Paul Smith

c.) The word happiness would lose its meaning if it weren't balanced by sadness.

d.) Happiness is a conscious choice, not an automatic response. ~Mildred Barthel

e.) The secret to being happy is accepting where you are in life and making the most of every single day.

f.) Happiness comes when we stop complaining about the problems we have and start thanking God for the blessings we do have.

## CHANGE YOUR MINDSET

I'd like to shift our thinking now the power of positive thinking. I am not going to throw a bunch of fluff at you, because I suffer from pain on a daily basis and know it is not easy, and some days not realistic. However, I would be doing this book and everyone reading it an injustice it if I didn't address the fact that there is unharnessed power in our mind we can use to our benefit.

I found some advice titled "6 Things that I had to give up in order to move forward." Again, please understand, we are all in a different place physically, mentally, and emotionally, so these are merely suggestions that I believe can help you change your mindset.

1. "I had to give up the idea that I was never going to be the same person again." If you think about it, we are all changing and growing over time anyway. I am not the same person I was 20 years ago, thankfully. We experience many life changes, marriage, divorce, having children, or becoming ill. So moving forward simply means accepting who we are. Say these words out loud to yourself: I am not the person I used to be, and I accept myself. This has helped me move forward.

2. "I had to stop beating myself up over my limitations." We are all unique individuals. Every single one of us has different limitations, thus there's no need to compare ourselves with one another. The weirdest part of this whole thing is that these limitations or differences are magnified when they are imposed or forced on us. It really is true that it seems we want something more when we know we cannot have it. Accepting the fact that we are all unique and special in our own way does not make you better or worse than anyone else. Be yourself, everyone else is already taken!

3. "I had to stop holding grudges." This was extremely hard for me because my grudge was against the Lord as well as other people I considered friends but who became too busy for me. While I do understand people have their jobs and expected them to have less time for me, I didn't expect to lose contact with them. These negative feelings began to grow into negative energy and anger which I finally realized was a complete waste of time and energy. I came across a powerful saying that helped me get past holding a grudge: "Holding a grudge is like drinking poison and waiting for the other person to die."

4. "I had to give up negativity." For those fighting chronic pain and illness, you already know this can be a daily battle. Negativity can include negative thought or negative people. Again, I came across some extreme words of wisdom that helped me move forward from the bad habit of thinking negative.

   a.) The less you respond to negativity, the more peaceful your life will become.

   b.) Negative thinking will never make your life positive.

   c.) Negative thinking destroys your brain cells. (Lord knows I cannot afford to lose any more brain cells than I already have.)

   d.) You cannot live a positive life with a negative mind.

   e.) Don't let your struggle become your identity. ~Toby Mac

   Moving on to address the negative people in your life, I have some other quotes from Pinterest that have helped me also change my perspective:

   a.) Don't let negative or toxic people rent the space in your head. Raise the rent and kick them out.

   b.) Stay away from negative people; they have a problem for every solution.

   c.) Your body hears everything your mind says, so stay positive.

   d.) If you care too much what other people think about you, you will always be their prisoner.

   e.) My life might not be going the way I planned it, but it's going the way God planned it.

5. "I had to stop wanting the life that others have." Remember the saying, "The grass always looks greener on the other side of the fence?" Well, that is not always the case. To sit and wish you have something others have forces you to be consumed with focusing on just the positive things you see in their life. When the truth is,

you really don't know what struggles that person has or the battles they are fighting. Take for example Joyce Meyer. She is a successful author, inspirational speaker, and sitting very well financially. I could sit and say, gee, I wish I had her life, which I used to do until I found out a few details about her life. She was consistently raped and molested not only by her father for many years, but other men as well. She was married to her first husband who ran around, drank, and left her pregnant and penniless. When she came home from the hospital she had no home to go to for her and her baby. She also survived through breast cancer. Upon reconsideration, I do not wish I had her life. Here are some quotes to give you food for thought.

a.) Envy is the art of counting other people's blessings instead of your own.

b.) Jealousy often grows from the root of low self-esteem.

c.) Be kind because everyone is fighting a battle you know nothing about.

6. "I had to stop worrying about what other people think." It's a waste of time and energy to consume yourself caring what other people think about you. It won't change the reality of your situation, but in fact, make you miserable. Think about these statements:

a.) It's not for us to judge the journey of anyone else's soul. You have to decide who you are and not care what anyone else thinks.

b.) It's not who you are that holds you back, it's who you think you are not.

c.) Just because my path is different doesn't mean I am lost.

d.) Be yourself: everyone else is already taken.

Reference: http://countingmyspoons.com/2015/11/6-things-that-i-had-to-give-up-in-order-to-move-forward/

## BE A PRISONER OF HOPE

Now we get to the heart and soul of this chapter. The "how" in the world do I turn my negative thoughts into positive ones. I'd like to say this has to be an intentional process. I know this because being ill and in pain, it's so easy to wake up wishing you hadn't. At many times in my life during the past several years I woke up only to find myself thinking, "Oh, I can tell this is going to be a bad day, I don't feel good, my pain is so bad today I won't be able to do anything and on and on." You may be saying, but I can't help what I think. Yes you can. Mentally place a stop sign up in your mind and chose to not let your mind dictate your thoughts. Whose mind is it? Who has control?

The question remains, how do we enjoy life despite our circumstances? It just so happens that I have some answers. Start with examining your thoughts that you wake up with each day and learn to identify self-defeating thoughts. We are often very harsh on ourselves within our self-talk. Ask yourself if the thoughts you are having accurate? This suspends the negativity for a moment and actually forces you to look for evidence to the contrary. If you write down your thoughts, it will put them at even more of a distance.

Since life does not come with a remote control we have to make a conscious choice to change our thoughts and chose to enjoy life to the best of our ability despite what we are going through. Sometimes that means one day at a time, one hour at a time, and sometimes one minute at a time. Sharing from my personal experience, my faith is what has carried me through all my storms and valleys of despair. I finally grabbed the bible verse "for I know the plans I have for you declares the Lord, plans to prosper and not harm you, plans to give you hope and a future" and used it as my foundation to stand upon Philippians 4:13.

Hope is a key factor in thinking positive. Hope can make the present moment less difficult to bear because if we believe that tomorrow will be better, we can bear the hardship of today. I once heard someone say, look back at all the difficult days you have endured. Your success rate is 100%, and they are right. If you stand your ground and do not give in to negative feelings, they will starve and lose power over us.

Quite honestly, there was a time that I felt my life was over and I was ready to go home and be with the Lord. My faith was my life jacket. I slowly started to listen to inspirational messages, and read scriptures from time to time. Then I came across an exciting verse where I was promised that God will give me double for my trouble (Isaiah 61:7). However, I was also reminded that a double blessing does not apply to someone who is double minded.

Living with FMS and chronic illness means our life is unpredictable from one day to the next, so the only way we can take any kind of charge of it, is by controlling and preparing our minds with a tool box so when the hard days come we are prepared to deal with it.

In order to not be led by my emotions, I had to have some major shifts in my thought paradigm. While I realize troubles, trials, doubt, fear, unbelief and plain weariness will come my way, my goal is to guard my mind and heart. The way I do that is by saying out loud that I will not let this defeat me and then as a believer I quote scripture out loud. I have actually said out loud, "Satan be gone. You are evicted from this address and from my life. You are no longer welcome in this home." Then I have a meeting with myself and give myself an attitude adjustment saying that life may not be everything I hoped it would be, but that I am blessed more than many people in this world. Then I start to start naming my blessings out loud or writing them down in my journal. It's funny how when we fill our minds with the right thoughts that the wrong ones have no room to enter ~Joyce Meyer

I have come across much research and strategies that can help anyone who makes a choice to give it a try. One of the first strategies is to simply admit you have FMS or whatever chronic illness you have. Do not pretend you are fine when you do not feel fine. This will help your loved ones around you also accept that this illness is real. A surprising piece of information I found is that when we avoid admitting to how bad we feel, that avoidance actually increases our fibro pain. So having an important outlet is key.

Keep a journal and write about your personal feelings. This is something I started doing a few years ago and it has helped me not only vent my feelings, but also keep track of events that occurred which has helped me identify triggers of my pain and fibro flares.

Have a positive attitude about your treatment. I have seen and heard this from many FMS patients. They tend to imprint their minds that fibro has completely devastated and hijacked their life. While it is true chronic illness and pain does change your life and abilities, there are still things we are able to do. In fact, helping others is the best way to take your mind off yourself. How is that possible you might ask? Well, in the months I was unable to drive and leave the house I decided to be a blessing to one person every day. I chose to send a card or letter, phone a friend, send someone a greeting through facebook or e-mail, give a hug, or encourage anyone that crossed my path. The other way you can encourage yourself is to talk to a counselor, read self-help books, or even join an online Facebook support group. I never knew they existed and when I ran across FAKS by accident. I sat in front of the computer as I read postings and cried because I realized I was not crazy and there were other people out there that felt like I did. I was no longer alone and this was my window to the outside world.

I'd like to share information from an article that discusses "Mental Shifts That Improved My Mental Health from **prohealth.com** written by Julie Ryan.

1. Change your "I cannot do it" mentality to "I can do it." This goes back to the old saying whether you believe you can't or you can, you are right. Tip: remember to be realistic.

2. "I cannot get by without _____" must be changed to "I don't really want ____ anyway." Fill in those blanks with whatever works for you. My choice would be foods that I really love like Italian food. I am working with a special doctor and have had to dramatically change my eating habits and I have come to realize that what I am gaining is worth so much more than what it's worth to sit and pig out on Italian or fast food.

3. "Health is supposed to be easy" has to become "Becoming healthly requires some work." Yes, I admit it. Just like many of you, I want a magic pill to take and make this weight disappear. While it is true that medications do contribute to the weight gain we suffer, I am here to personally testify that I am on steroids (which causes weight gain) and will have to be for the rest of my life. Yet with discipline, work, and dedication I am losing weight. I might also add that Gabipentin is another medication famously known for weight gain. I am on that too. So yes, it can be done. I will explain more in depth in the next chapter regarding the program I am working on with my functional medicine doctor.

4. "I can't do it now" has to change to "Now is the best time to get it done." Procrastinating until tomorrow means tomorrow will never come. Remember the definition of insanity is doing the same thing and expecting different results. In order to be successful in no matter the task, you have to begin today.

5. Fitting nicely with the above information are the tips given by a fellow FM patient who says to focus on the 4 P's:

   a.) Pacing yourself

   b.) Problem solving

c.) Prioritizing

d.) Planning

6.  Accept your limits. We all have good days and bad days. On a good day set a few realistic goals while remembering to pace yourself. On a bad day, set ONE goal for yourself. That one goal might be to simply get out of bed. It might be to take a shower. I have had many days when I know it was going to take every ounce of energy to just take a shower and that was using my shower chair. I hated that I was only 43 and needed to use a shower chair, but decided that I would rather not fall in the shower and hit my head or get hurt. So be realistic, pace your activities, prioritize, and plan to set goals.

Since you already know negative thoughts can re-wire your brain, let's discuss the fact that positive thinking can also do the same thing. Because of the biochemical link between the mind and body, it makes sense that positive thoughts, feelings, and optimism will reduce levels of stress hormones thereby reducing stress. It also stimulates the part of the nervous system responsible for slowing heartrate, intestinal and glandular activities.

The re-wiring of the brain does not take place automatically but through a series of practice and steps. The first thing required is that you have to learn to love yourself. Next you need to respect the journey. In an ideal world, you need to practice these steps that will indeed lead to re-wiring your brain to replace negative thoughts with positive ones. Here are the 5 steps as follows:

7.  Be Aware:

a.) Recognize the triggers of your negative thoughts and when they are occurring.

b.) Like the layers of an onion, allow yourself time to peel layers back in an effort to identify the negative influences in and on your life.

c.) Allow yourself time and compassion to change your thoughts.

d.) Be aware of the benefits this will bring to you which may be a strong motivator.

e.) Make sure your worst enemy is not living between your two ears. ~Don Loyd

8. Take responsibility for your actions:

   a.) Remember that humans have an average of 70,000 thoughts a day.

   b.) Admit you can have control over your thoughts.

   c.) If you have given others control of your thought life, start by taking it back a little at a time.

   d.) Set boundaries for those trying to control your thoughts.

   e.) We cannot solve our problems with the same thinking we used when we created them. ~Albert Einstein

9. Make a Plan

   a.) Start every single day with a plan to recite a positive statement, prayer, or affirmation.

   b.) Affirmations are positive personalized statements with a desired goal or outcome.

   c.) Examples of positive affirmations might include: I chose to be happy, I give myself permission to take a nap today without feeling guilty, I am choosing to say no today because I don't feel well enough to go out as planned, I will no longer allow people to make me feel guilty, I am thankful for what I have, I am going to count my blessings, I deserve to be happy.

   d.) Set at least one goal for the day. Examples might include: I will read a book today, I am going to take a nap today, I will do the dishes today, I will take a shower. Whatever you chose keep in mind what your limitations are.

e.) This is your personal time. Choose to do something that makes you happy.

10. Practice, Practice, Practice:

a.) Continue your positive affirmations every single day.

a.) Repetition activates, chemical processes that re-wire your brain and set a positive attitude, and breaks down new pathways for positive thinking.

b.) Practice replacing negative talk with positive thoughts:

| Negative self-talk | Positive self-talk |
|---|---|
| I have never tried this before | This is a chance for me to learn something new |
| It's too difficult | Let me look at this from a new standpoint |
| It's impossible. This will never work | I am going to try to make it work |
| I'm no good at this | I'll try again |

ENJOY!

a.) Remember that as the brain re-wires itself your health will improve.

b.) Better health= a better life.

## TAKE YOUR PICK

Let's conclude this section and begin the next one with a chart that shows comparisons between positive and negative thinking. I encourage you to examine each column and then, take your pick as to which you would prefer.

| Effects of Negative Thinking | Effects of Positive Thinking |
|---|---|
| 1. Prolonged wound healing | 1. Decreased pain |
| 2. Frequent respiratory infections | 2. Better sleep |
| 3. Infections in general | 3. Strengthens the immune system |
| 4. Headaches/migraines | 4. Increased sense of well being |
| 5. Muscle twitches and fatigue | 5. Quicker healing |
| 6. Alienation | 6. Reduced cardiac disease |
| 7. Irritability | 7. Optimistic |
| 8. Insomnia | 8. Lower cholesterol and blood pressure |
| 9. Accident prone | 9. Less pain |
| 10. Loss of sex drive | 10. Improves breathing |
| 11. Impaired judgement | 11. Improves sex life |
| 12. Fatigue | 12. Less joint pain |
| 13. Loss of confidence | 13. Less back pain |
| 14. Negativity | 14. More confidence |
| 15. Development of bad habits-drinking, drugs | 15. More motivation |
| 16. Ulcers | 16. Creative |
| 17. High blood pressure | 17. Loving |
| 18. Heart attacks | 18. More energy |
| 19. Chest pain | 19. Helps us reach our goals |
|  | 20. Overall happier |

There are many other steps that will help you live with FM or chronic illness. I will share some of the ones that have helped me. Additionally, at the end of the chapter I will include a list of resources so you can investigate more on your own time. One of the biggest shifts in my life was when I took a personal vow to not let fibro control me. I realized that I was just existing and not living. Granted, there are still days that pain limits me, but those are the days my goals are small, and that is ok. I still look at the overall picture of my life as I might have fibro, but it does not have me.

This leads easily to the next concept of understanding that there will be days that are better than others. The key is to be sure you make that personal vow to now give up or let yourself feel defeated. Do what you can on those days and let the rest go. I came across a statement that has helped me significantly which reads: I need to be able to say no today, without feeling guilty. So do you!

## ADDITIONAL TOOLS

Find a support system. Be sure to maximize all of your resources. Some support systems include family and friends; however, not everyone has that luxury. You might need to find an actual fibro support group you can attend in your area. I know when I found the fibromyalgia support group on Facebook, I was so relieved to be able to identify with a group of people that actually felt the same way physically, emotionally, and mentally that I did. I grew and continue to grow to care so much about multiple people in this group that I consider some of these folks a second family. I have become part of the administrative team which means I have committed and taken a leadership role in the group. It gives me deep satisfaction to know that I can be a light in a world of pain for people that may need help or otherwise might have no support system.

Speaking of support systems, have you thought about a service dog or pet? Your doctor has to write a note for medical needs or the need for emotional support and the cost of the animal and maintenance can be written off on federal taxes. This information comes from someone who owns a service animal. At the end of the chapter, I will include some reference sites for you to get more information on the subject.

Absolutely do not focus on what you cannot do. Focus on what you can do. I guarantee that when you focus on your inabilities they become even bigger obstacles. I bet each and every one of us can identify with the saying "Every day I engage in a wrestling match between what I want to do, and what I can do." However at the end of the night, be OK with what it is that you were actually able to complete. Keep your sense of perspective; when things become overwhelming, take a step back. Sometimes there are reasons you feel this way including fatigue, a severe lack of sleep, and pain. When your eyes become fixed on your inabilities we seem to fall into a pit of despair. Once in the pit, it is very hard to dig your way out.

Decrease your level of stress. It's a fact that life brings on certain stresses we cannot control. However, there are many things that are in our control. Do not overcommit yourself. Don't say yes to an activity or event when your heart and mind are screaming "NO, I can't do it."

EDUCATE YOURSELF! Remember knowledge is power. I found that the more I increased my knowledge the better equipped and more self-confident I was when I walked into a physician's office. The other thing education did for me was boost my sense of self-worth. It was actually when I started living instead of feeling like I was just surviving or existing from one day to the next.

A caveat to educating yourself is to educate others as to when you are hurting or not feeling well. Many people do not know that it hurts us to be touched. We have to let them know. So tell them that you would rather have a high five as opposed to a hug, because right now a hug would hurt. If you are the type of person that doesn't want people to ask you how you feel, simply tell them that and add because you'd rather not focus on that right now.

Dealing with chronic pain and illness can be downright exhausting. We have to grant ourselves permission to be tired, weak, and in pain.

Remember, you are allowed to cry and scream, but you are not allowed to give up. For those of us who have faith in God, giving up means that you are saying that the enemy is stronger than our Lord. Faith has kept me alive and determined that I will not let this illness define who I am.

Laughter is the best medicine, use humor throughout the day. Happiness, smiling, and laughing help your body produce endorphins and healthy chemicals which are natural pain and stress relievers. Something I learned when reading about endorphins is that they trigger feelings in your body similar to that of morphine. Here are some natural ways to increase your endorphins. **(http://www.rd.com/health/8-ways-to-naturally-increase-endorphins/)**

a.) Smell the scent of vanilla or lavender- which also helps depression and insomnia. "According to a study at the Memorial Sloan-Kettering Cancer Center, patients undergoing MRIs who breathed vanilla-scented air reported 63 percent less anxiety than those who breathed unscented air." **(rd.com)**

b.) Take Ginseng which has also shown to improve memory and concentration.

c.) Exercise to the best of your ability. There were some days the only thing I could do was sit on the couch and do leg lifts from the edge of the couch. When I was so weak and mostly bedbound, I asked my physician if I could have home physical therapy (PT). When I was working with PT I was discouraged because I could no longer walk 20 minutes on my treadmill like I could at one time. They told me not to worry about it. Start with one minute walks then stop. Then I could build up to 2 minutes and so on. I am now up to 10 minutes at a time, and I am keeping a positive attitude because I am making forward progress. Exercise does not have to mean you go jogging, run a marathon, or sign up for an aerobics. Everyone knows their physical limitations, so remember that and just get your body moving the best you can.

d.) LAUGHTER! Again, we come across the importance and benefits of laughter. Did you know that children laugh on an average of 300 times a day and adults laugh approximately five times a day? Neither did I. "Laughter is sometimes described as 'inner jogging'. Research has shown that it can help to: lower blood pressure, reduce stress hormones, boost immune function by raising levels of infection-fighting cells,trigger the release of endorphins, the body's natural painkillers. and produce a general sense of well-being." **(http://www.rd.com/health/8-ways-to-naturally-increase-endorphins/).**

## POSITIVE ASPECTS OF FM

The last subject I'd like to speak about is the Positive aspects of fibromyalgia. I saved this statement for last because some of you might think I have fallen and received a head injury. No, I have not. I have collected a combination of resources and when I start feeling down and out, I pull my resources, sayings, poems, or words of encouragement and they help me tremendously.

I'd like to start with a few positive affirmation statements:

a.) I never knew pain until fibromyalgia knocked me down. I never knew strength until I got back up. I am a fibro WARRIOR. (Facebook.com/fibrocolors)

b.) I am not fibromyalgia. I am what kicks its butt every morning when I get out of bed.

c.) Don't be ashamed of your story; it will inspire others.

d.) I don't want my pain and struggle to make me a victim. I want my battle to make me someone else's hero.

e.) I want to inspire people. I want someone to look at me and say, "Because of you, I didn't give up."

f.) Who can I be a blessing to today?

g.) I love and approve of myself.

h.) Every day may not be good, but there is something good in every day.

i.) It is enough to do my best.

j.) Greater is He that is in me than he that is in the world. 1John 4:4

k.) I can do all things through Christ who gives me strength Philippians. 4:13

l.) Trust in the Lord with all your heart, lean not on your own understanding. In all your ways acknowledge Him, and He will direct your paths. Proverbs 3:5-6

m.) The joy of the Lord is my strength. Nehemiah 8:10

n.) Don't believe everything you think.

o.) Faith is the only thing I know that is stronger than fear.

p.) Worry is a down payment on a problem you may never have. ~Joyce Meyer

q.) Where ever you go, leave a heart print.

r.) The soul would have no rainbows if the eyes had no tears. ~Native American Proverb

s.) We are stronger in the places we have been broken. ~Ernest Hemingway

ONE of my Favorites:

a.) We learn through our brokenness what we could never learn through our wholeness. ~Dr. David Jeremiah

Now that I have shared with you some personal quotes that help me focus on the silver lining during my cloudy days, I want to share just a few more ideas before concluding this chapter. Finding the good side of fibromyalgia probably sounds like a paradox to you. However, as I said above, I really do believe there is something positive we can find in every situation.

Fibro forces a person to find out what you are really made of, or find your inner strength. There are days when you want to give up, yet there are days you wake up and see the sunshine and realize it's a new day to count your blessings. Strength doesn't come from doing things you know you can do, but overcoming things you thought you couldn't. Did you know that trials often come our way not to discover our weaknesses, but to discover our inner strength?

When you have an illness, it allows you to empathize with others and help them. It's easy to say the words 'I know how you feel', which is ignorance unless you have walked a mile in their shoes. There is so much truth to that saying. I have found courage and strength from making the best out of my illness. I am helping others by being a light that shines in the darkness, being an encouragement to others, and just listening to people vent. I told myself that I had find a purpose for my pain. I want to make this test, my testimony, this mess my message, and change from being a victim to having victory.

This illness has taught me an incredibly valuable lesson in life that many people never learn which is what is most important in life. Like many others I had aspirations for many things. However, I have come to realize the most important things in life are not possessions or money. As a student nurse I read a story written by a doctor about a man who was dying. At the end of one's life he said he had never had a patient ask for their financial portfolio to be brought in, nor their fancy car, or even a valuable collection of coins. However, what people do want near the end of their life is family and/or loved ones.

To piggyback off what is genuinely important in life, I have learned that having a spotless house isn't more important than snuggling with my daughter, taking and appreciating pictures of the sunrises, sunsets, or nature which has become a big part of my life. I never realized how much I took advantage of the little things in life, until I became ill.

You see, many people take it for granted and just jump in their car when they want to go to the store, rush through the day and without recognizing when someone is sad or needs an encouraging word. Acts 20:35 says "It is better to give than to receive." I have found that to be so true. It is satisfying to the soul when you can bless someone especially when you are going through your own storm. It takes the focus off myself when I help others. (fibromyalgia.newlifeoutlook.com)

Here are some specific suggestions to shine brighter and help maintain your confidence when suffering from chronic illness or pain. As previously mentioned, it is easy to look to the dark side of chronic illness which often triggers a lower self-esteem. Depression will minimize your achievements, but thinking on the following will help magnify the positive. Things to focus on include the following:

a.) What is your gift or talent? We all have special gifts and just be-cause we have acquired an illness does not mean we have to let it completely steal it from us.

b.) Describe your character. Think of explanative words or phrases that describe your personality and focus on those positive qual-ities.

c.) Recall past successes in your life. We all have personal value and contributions we have made to society, family, or our own lives. It might take some effort because chronic illness likes to steal your joy, but I bet if you give this some time and thought you can focus on how you have helped this world become a better place. Don't discount anything meaning, making new friends, being able to at-tend a bible study, or just make it to all your doctor appointments within the past year. It all counts.

d.) What is your most immediate goal? As discussed earlier, it's important to have a goal, no matter how big or small it may seem to you. Accomplishments help boost your self-esteem.

e.) What is your biggest mistake and what did you learn from it? Don't dwell on mistakes but when you ignore them it means you cannot learn from them. Here are a few quotes to remember:

1. You can learn great things when you aren't busy ignoring them.

2. Mistakes are stepping stones to learning.

3. Mistakes have the power to turn you into something better than you were before. ~KushandWizdom

4. Your mistakes do not define you.

5. Life is all about making choices, always do your best to make the right ones, and always learn your best to learn from the wrong ones. - *unknown*

## WHAT CAN I DO?

Lastly, I'd like to share a few ideas to occupy yourself when you find yourself with too much time on your hands. I have noticed a tendency to focus on my problems until they just grow and grow and nothing else seemed to matter. My mind was so pre-occupied on my inabilities and illness that I didn't have room or time for anything else. I have had other people ask the question of me, "I have so much time on my hands because I cannot work, so what can I do with myself?" I found myself compiling a list to share and keep for myself. This is by no means all inclusive, but at least there are some references to get you started in getting your mind off yourself:

1. Play in the dirt!

* Dirt makes you naturally happy because it contains natural anti-

depressant microbes called Mycobacterium vaccae, which has the same effect as Prozac.

» It also stimulates serotonin production which helps make us happy and calm.

» Studies were actually conducted on cancer patients who reported less stress and a higher quality of life.

» This microbe is also being studies for its effects on rheumatoid arthritis, mental functions and even Chron's disease. **(gardening-knowhow.com)**

2. Go to You-tube and pick some inspirational messages to listen to from Joyce Meyer, Joel Olsteen, Charles Stanley, or a favorite evangelist you may know and like.

3. Listen to uplifting music.

4. Go for a walk- if you are able.

5. Send a card to a friend you haven't seen or talked to in a while.

6. Send a card to a sick friend.

7. Perform a random act of kindness.

8. Pick up your bible—look in the concordance—and pick a subject you know you need to work on and read scripture.

9. Read "The Battlefield of the Mind" by Joyce Meyer- one of my favorite books.

10. Go to Youtube and find some FUNNY videos to watch...LAUGH! It's good for the soul. I used to love the show "Whose line is it anyway" which is a very funny show and always made me laugh. I found some clips on You Tube and would sit and laugh, and I always feel better after laughing. I bet you will too. Find some bloopers on Youtube—anything funny.

11. Write a letter to family, friends, or anyone you feel angry at then BURN IT.

12. Go to this web site and read it: **http://www.lifehack.org/articles/life-style/10-ways-cheer-yourself-when-youre-bad-mood.html**

13. Watch a funny movie.

14. Look at positive/inspirational quotes.

15. Write in a journal.

16. Hug someone.

17. Have some chocolate.

18. Let it out. Cry your eyes out if you need to – it reduces tension and will help you feel better. Just don't let it go on too long! It's only healthy to wallow in your feelings for a little while.

19. Look at blue. According to color psychology, looking at the color blue relaxes your mind. Studies have yet to back this up, but hey, it can't hurt, right? If you hate blue, try another color that puts you in a good mood –like light pinks or greens.

20. COLOR a picture! Yes that's right. They make adult stress relieving coloring books you can get most anywhere. I use gel pens because it easier to get in those small spaces. Here is an example of a pic I colored. It was actually fun and got my mind off myself.To see images in color, please see my web site **www.kellyhemingway.com**

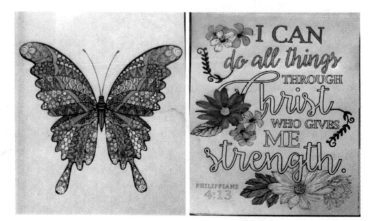

21. Speed up your thinking. A 2009 study showed that thinking quickly makes you feel more powerful, energetic and happy. So how do you do that? Try imposing a time limit on solving a riddle, or watch a movie in fast-forward.

22. Take a nap.

23. Meditate for 15 minutes.

24. Go outside and get some fresh air.

25. Paint a picture. Be creative. Jamie Buchanan from CT, had brain cancer and chemo therapy which led to fibromyalgia. Jamie has offered to share her talent with us. To see images in color, please see my web site **www.kellyhemingway.com**
    Thanks for sharing Jamie.

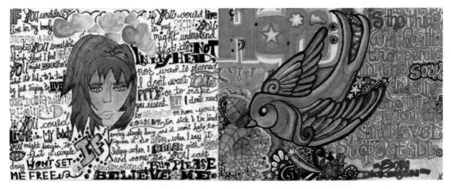

26. Exercise Your Brain

    Just like our body needs exercise, so does our brain! Try doing a little each day using a combination of brainteasers, crossword puzzles, or whatever you enjoy.

27. Try to limit stress in your life

    Stress can exacerbate fibro symptoms. Though it's impossible to avoid any stress in your life, there are ways to help deal with life:

» Take regular breaks from work and home life.

» Reduce your workload.

» Practice meditation.

» Get regular exercise to help deal with excess energy or stressful situations.

28. Breathing correctly:

Lie down on your back in a comfortable position.

Place your hand on your stomach, just below your belly button.

Take a deep breath in through your nose and hold it for a moment.

Slowly exhale, through your nose.

When you think you have let out all of the air, open your mouth and let the rest out.

When you breathe "from the belly" and use your diaphragm, your body gets more oxygen and can get rid of more built up waste gases.

**http://www.fibromyalgia-symptoms.org/fibromyalgia_memory_loss.html**

29. Read!

One of my favorite books that helped me perceive chronic illness from a different perspective: *The Sweet Side of Suffering by M. Esther Lovejoy*. Its only $10.00 on **Amazon.com**.

In conclusion, the connection between the mind and body has an immense effect on our entire state of well-being. Every day we wake up there is a choice to think positive or negative. Remember, even if you are having a rough day, admit and allow yourself to feel the pain and give yourself permission to say no and rest for the day. There are multiple things we can do to help ourselves whether it's consciously or subconsciously. My hope is that I have helped you see things from a slightly different perspective and consider the power of the mind.

Here are some web sites for service pet information

1. http://usdogregistry.org/?gclid=CNnShP-coMwCFZGIaQod-mMD7g

2. http://usdogregistry.org/information/information-on-service-dogs/

3. https://adata.org/publication/service-animals-booklet

4. http://www.therapydoginfo.net/servicedogs.html

5. https://invisibledisabilities.org/connect/onlineresources/serviceanimalin-fo/

# CHAPTER 5

## HELP YOURSELF

*Give Thanks for what you are now and keep fighting*
*for what you want to be tomorrow*

*Fernanda Miramontes-Landeros*

I'd like to begin this chapter by saying there is no way humanly possible I can cover every single type of medication, treatment, supplement, or homeopathic treatment used for chronic illness and pain. I will, however, try and hit the ones most commonly discussed among the specialists. Additionally, I want to re-iterate that I am in no way advocating any treatment, as I am not a physician. I just want to bring information to the forefront that is helping people all over the United States and the world.

### FUNCTIONAL VERSUS TRADITIONAL MEDICINE

Functional Medicine is a term I have become familiar with just within the past year or so. In the world of medicine it is being hailed as the up and coming trend in medicine because chronic illness has become a plague in this country and in the world. Over 125 million Americans are affected by chronic diseases (mindbodygreen.com).

At this time I'd like to differentiate between traditional and functional medicine as well as provide multiple ways you can take some control back from the chronic pain that is controlling you. That's right. You have multiple ways you can help yourself. Before you decide to skip this chapter because you think I am going to preach about diet and exercise, although I will discuss it, I'd like to educate and empower you with some awesome information: "Knowledge is Power!"

Traditional versus Functional Medicine, I have put some characteristics in a comparative chart. Prior to discussing the underlying problems in chronic pain, illness and fibromyalgia, I'd like to inject a bit of humor but with total truth being told. These statements come from Dr. Roger Murphree, the Fibro Doctor, and functional medicine doctor, who has treated FM for approximately 20 years. His book is called *Treating and Beating Fibromyalgia & Chronic Fatigue Syndrome*. I actually laughed out loud when I read the following statements found in his book.

You might have a stupid doctor if:

1. They tell you fibromyalgia does not exist.

2. They dismiss your symptoms because you want attention.

3. It's all in your mind.

4. You are a hypochondriac.

5. They tell you to exercise more, eat healthier, lose weight.

6. You are just depressed.

7. Your blood work is completely normal thus labeling you as a drug-seeker even though you never asked for it.

8. They refuse to order proper tests, especially a thyroid test, test for adrenal fatigue because of the constant pain which causes stress

and drains your adrenal glands-among other tests. This is why it is so important to educate yourself, you need to be able to ask questions as to why they are not ordering the appropriate tests.

9.   They have you taking a drug that stimulates and relaxes you. Some of these meds are addictive. Doctors like to overmedicate patients to control symptoms, not fix the problem.

Many if not all of you will identify with the basic fact that traditional medicine focuses on your specific problem and drugs that match the symptoms or disease. I have personally been on at least 75-100 different medications within the past 6 years because doctors couldn't find the right medication to help me. Sometimes my symptoms would subside but then I would develop side effects which required another medication to counteract the one they gave me. I felt like a toxic waste dump. It became nothing more than a viscous cycle that I finally got fed up with, thus I looked for an alternative method and doctor to help me. Examine in the chart below, the difference between traditional versus functional medicine.

| Traditional Medicine Focus | Functional Medicine Focus |
| --- | --- |
| Lacks the perspective or knowledge to look for underlying causes | Search for underlying or root cause of problem |
| Looks at the set of symptoms and asks what drugs or hormones match this disease or symptoms | Searches for why patient has the problem, why function has been lost, and asks HOW function can be restored, searches for underlying cause |
| Addresses and usually focuses on a set of symptoms or disease | Addresses the patient as a whole and has a team approach when developing care |
| Oriented towards acute care | Tailors treatment to the patient's individual and unique needs |
| Lacks tools for preventing chronic illness or underlying cause of diseases | Promotes health and concerned with more than just the absence of disease |
| Prescription meds are the standard of care model that is used | Supports the fact that our body has internal mechanisms to heal itself |

| | |
|---|---|
| Often refers to specialist for specific system disease processes-who generally focus on the specific organ or system, not the person as a whole | Assesses patient's internal and external environment. Treats patient holistically, mind, body and soul |
| Huge gap in research and practice | Trained to consider the origin, prevention and treatment of chronic diseases |
| Fails miserably as evidenced by the growing epidemic of chronic illness (125 million) and the rising cost of healthcare | Integration of traditional and alternative treatments which might include: medications, natural supplements, specific lab testing or diagnostics, herbal supplements, or homeopathic alternatives |

*Source (mindbodygreen.com)*

## PRESCRIPTION & OVER THE COUNTER MEDS

Let's start with something we are all familiar with, prescription medications. I will focus on the prescription medications that have been approved by the FDA to treat FMS. Please understand since fibro folks often suffer from additional conditions, it usually takes a combination of meds to help relieve symptoms; The current approved meds to treat fibro meds are Lyrica (pregabalin), Cymbalta (duloxetine hydrochloride) and Savella (milnacipran HCL). All are supposed to be able to reduce pain but the mechanism of action is unclear. All have side effects that can mimic the symptoms of fibromyalgia. Personally speaking, I have been on all three of these medications and suffered some severe side effects, some of which put me in the hospital. However, I would like to remind everyone that we are all individuals and I have heard testimonies from people who take these meds and they have helped the pain and ability to function.

There are other medications, doctors use to treat FMS, including Neurotonin (gabapentin) which is a med used to treat seizures and nerve pain. This happens to be the medication I am currently taking and it has been effective in helping to decrease my pain. The problem for me, as well as many others I have spoken to, is weight gain.

As a word of caution, many of these medications have the same side effects of FMS. I have read some very concerning information regarding how many of these drugs have been pushed through the system. Just a few examples of this include Warner-Lambert sending physicians to an all-expense paid weekend at a plush resort, paying educational systems to create scientific articles to support their drug, paying physicians for each patient they agreed to put on a drug trial delaying publication and withholding information that could damage the marketing of a drug. I was appalled to find out that in 2004 Pfizer pled guilty for fraudulently marketing Neurotonin for unapproved uses. This information has put some serious doubt in my mind when it comes to trusting medications. (*Treating and Beating Fibromyalgia & Chronic Fatigue Syndrome,* Dr Roger Murphree, 2013).

Analgesics such as Ibuprofen, aspirin and Tylenol are the most common ones used. It's hard for me to not laugh at the thought of trying this to control pain. I would compare taking these meds to taking a sugar pill; absolutely ineffective. I only have one kidney, so I am unable to take Ibuprofen or meds comparable to it. Be careful with these meds they can cause GI (gastrointestinal) upset and bleeds.

Other pain meds that might be considered are Tramadol which requires a prescription. Please be aware that every medication I list has multiple side effects, so educate yourself when you are prescribed any medication so you know what to be looking out for.

I'd like to specifically mention the drug category Opioids which include: Vicodin, Percocet, OxyContin, and Codeine to name a few. According to Dr. Clauw's research that compared a fibro brain to a healthy patient's brain, the fibro patient has fewer opioid receptors in their brain to receive the med and allow it to help relieve pain. In simple terms, visualize receptor cells in the brain as a lock and opioid meds as a key. So if one pill represents 10 keys and it travels to the brain and finds only three locks, the other seven keys will float uselessly because there is no receptor(or lock) to unlock and allow it to work; thus providing the patient with ineffective pain relief.

Other medications that might be considered:

1. Muscle relaxers: reduce pain and muscle soreness, possibly help to sleep.

   Examples include: Soma, Flexeril, Skelaxin, Robaxin

2. Benzodiazepines: a group of medications that supports sleep relaxes muscles and helps anxiety. Be aware they cause drowsiness and can be addictive.

   Examples: Xanax, Restoril, Valium, Klonopin

3. Sleeping Pills: fibro and chronic pain sufferers have poor sleep patterns and we all know how important sleep is to help the body function properly.

   Examples: Ambien, Sonota, Lunesta

4. Antidepressants: chronic illness affects our brain chemicals causing an imbalance. There's no need to be ashamed of admitting you need an anti-depressant. Although I will admit, I resisted the idea for a while because I didn't want to be considered crazy or psycho. However, after my physician, whom had also been a colleague while I was a practicing nurse, told me that after all the hell I'd been through, anyone would need help coping, I decided to give in.

   Examples: Zoloft, Celexa, Buproprion, and many more

There are multiple other prescription meds that I cannot fully incorporate within the scope of this book. However, I will mention the categories and strongly advise that you always educate yourself as to the side effects. Other categories include Selective Serotonin Reuptake Inhibitors (SSRI's), Tricyclic antidepressants (TCA's).

Another medication I'd like to mention that seems to be getting more attention is called Low Dose Naltrexone or LDN. According to **http:// www.lowdosenaltrexone.org/** this medication is FDA approved. In low doses it helps fortify the immune system and helps with the following medical diagnoses: HIV/AIDS, cancer, autoimmune diseases such as lupus and rheumatoid arthritis, fibromyalgia, irritable bowel syndrome, Chrons, central nervous system disorders, and much much more. It does require a physician prescription.

I came across some very encouraging information at ldnresearchtrust. org, whose founder is Linda Elsegood who lives in the United Kingdom. Linda Elsegood says LDN has given her life back to her. She suffers from multiple sclerosis and was wheelchair bound as well as incontinent of her bowel and bladder. She also said she had lost most of her hearing and sight. After 18 months of LDN, she was able to walk and most every single one of her symptoms was reversed.

She warns that some doctors may not want to prescribe it because there is not much scientific research on it, it can be difficult to get, doctors don't want to think outside the box, and some just don't want to make time to research it. Her suggestion: research it yourself, talk to your doctor about prescribing it, and if they won't, find a different doctor who will.

A growing number of patients are finding relief with LDN, including a woman from Michigan who had tried everything she thought was possible. She said her leg pain was so bad she wanted to cut them off. She was ready to give up until seeing LDN on the Dr. Oz show. After approximately six weeks not only was her pain significantly improved but her depression and brain fog lifted and her memory also improved.

LDN is thought to work by having an anti-inflammatory effect on the brain. There's a special group of cells, microglial cells, in the brain that search for problems in the central nervous system, or CNS (brain and spinal cord). When they find abnormalities such as inflammation, the CNS thinks you have an infection and chemicals are released that cause pain, fatigue, and interference with thought processes. So it is thought that the LDN calms those microglial brain cells, thereby reducing inflammation and all the symptoms associated with it. Lastly, I'd like to mention that it is said that approximately 65% of people taking LDN benefit from a decrease in their overall symptoms. Unfortunately, LDN is not legal in all 50 states.

As I sit here and type, I wanted to share with you that after speaking with multiple physicians a specialty pharmacist named Michael Collins who was recently awarded National Pharmacist of the Year, I decided to wean off my narcotics I was taking for back pain and try LDN. I sit in amazement because my back pain is finally tolerable. I have been getting steroid injections into my back every two months or so because I have 3 pinched nerves, sciatica (sciatic nerve pain that runs down my leg so bad I can hardly walk), and spinal stenosis. My mobility was hindered as well as my quality of life due to extreme back pain. At this point in time I have been on LDN for 2 weeks and my pain has decreased from 8/10 down to 3/10. I also like the fact that LDN helps build the immune system by helping the body produce more helper-T cells, which are of major important to our immune system. Because it strengthens our immune system, LDN is also useful for those of us with autoimmune diseases. I am praying I can get off my Humira injections I take for my rheumatoid arthritis. For more information regarding LDN you can go to ldnresearchtrust.org or mercola.com.

Something important for you to be aware of about LDN is that it has a stigma attached to it. What does that mean? LDN, at much higher doses, is used to treat opioid withdrawal. Thus if you go to the ER and they see you are on LDN you could be labeled as a drug seeker. However, this is a GREAT time to educate them that this is not the case because LDN dosage for opioid withdrawal is 50-200mg. Your dosage is likely to range between 1.5-4.5 for fibromyalgia or other pain control issues.

## MEDICAL MARIJUANA

Morgan Freeman, a famous actor, is known in the fibro world as a strong advocate for medical marijuana. There are multiple articles posted within our fibro FB group where Morgan Freeman says that this is what allows him to continue to live his life productively.

In an article titled "Medical Marijuana: Top 10 Pros and Cons," there are opinions posted from a doctor's perspective, medical organizations, the US government views, its addictiveness and the gateway effect, among other issues. As I read through the article I found that basically under each of the Pro columns, there was a con to counter every pro reason provided. For example, under the addictiveness column, the pros listed were that there is very little evidence to support it's a true addiction and that there are no withdrawal symptoms. Under the con column, it states just the opposite and says there are withdrawal affects similar to that of nicotine. If you wish to read more info regarding this article you can find it at **ProCon.org.**

I want to be sure everyone understands there are multiple forms medical marijuana can take including: marinol which is a pill, the type you can smoke, cannabidiols (CBD) oil, brewed as tea, or as liquids vaporized into e-cigarettes. Medical marijuana is not legal in every state. I'd like to end this subject on a note that everyone has the choice to treat their symptoms as they wish, however, if you wish to "get healthy," this is not the way to do it.

## KRATOM

This is a medicinal plant native to Southeast Asia. Apparently it is extremely effective for pain. Some fibro folks in my online FB support group say that Kratom gave them their life back. Some sources say Kratom is highly addictive, others say it is not. There are multiple uses for Kratom including but not limited to: pain relief, energy production, depression, anti-inflammatory, and fighting anxiety. I will list some web sites for reference at the end of this chapter if you would like to investigate further **(Toptenz.net)** & **(speciose.org).**

With that being said, my experience in taking some of the medications commonly prescribed for fibro is like putting a Band-Aid on a bleeding artery . Yes, medications can be helpful, and even necessary in particular cases, but they do not make a person healthy. I want to say that everyone has free-will and has the choice to do what they feel is best for them. Not every solution is going to be the same for any particular individual. However, if you have the chance to fix the underlying problem, wouldn't you like that opportunity?

## COMMON DEFICIENCIES

There are a number of common deficiencies/problems that are specific to FMS, some of which include: energy, serotonin, magnesium, Vitamin B-12, adrenal hormone (cortisol, DHEA), and vitamin D. See the chart below for ways to naturally help each of the issues just mentioned.

Having a basic understanding of the following information will enable you to not only understand WHY some of the following natural supplements, herbs, and foods will help, but it will explain WHY you are medically experiencing some of the problems you have. After reading the slides below, I bet you will be able to easily identify multiple symptoms you have related to the function of each nutrient

Think back to the leaky gut syndrome and how it allows multiple undigested nutrients and bacteria out into the bloodstream and body as discussed in chapter one. Many fibro folks are deficient in multiple nutrients because they never have the chance to be properly absorbed. I'd like you to understand the importance of a few neurotransmitters and chemicals that are essential to those of us with fibro or chronic illness. Most serotonin is found in the brain, bowels and blood platelets. The function of it is to communicate messages between nerve cells, regulate many body processes; serotonin can affect mood and social behavior, appetite and digestion, sleep, memory and sexual desire and function, and helps maintain a sense of wellbeing and happiness. It is vital for mood balance and researchers believe that a lack of serotonin leads to depression. (http://www.medicalnewstoday.com/articles/232248.php).

## Adrenal Gland Hormones

- STRESS Response
- Helps control blood sugar & blood pressure
- Helps regulate metabolism
- Produce aprox 50 different hormones
- Fights allergens, infections, auto-immune diseases
- Converts food for energy
- Important for a healthy heart
- Sex drive
- Essential to your overall health
- Anti-inflammatory
- http://www.adrenalfatigue.co.nz/adrenal-gland-function/
- Pic: re

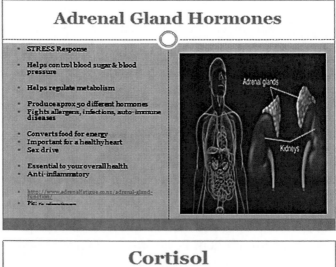

## Cortisol

- Produced by adrenal gland
- Helps with:
*Body's stress response
*Regulate blood pressure
*Slows inflammatory process
*Helps insulin break down
    sugar for energy use
*Regulates metabolism

https://pituitary.org/knowledge-base/disorders/adrenal-insufficiency-addison-s-disease).

Pic: newresolvehypnosis.com

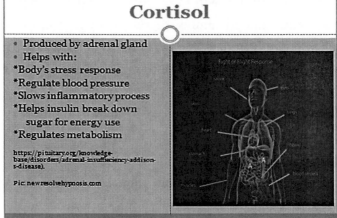

## DHEA (dehydroepiandrosterone)

- Produced by adrenal gland
- Provides energy
- Helps immune system
- Improves mood
- Improves memory
- Improves mental function
- Improves sexual function
- Muscle strength
- Bone building
- 2011 International Society for Sexual Medicine.
- Pic: humananatomybody.info

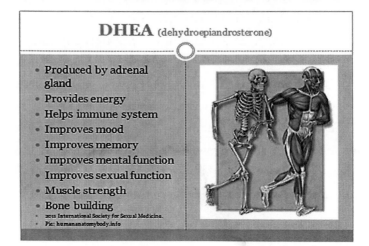

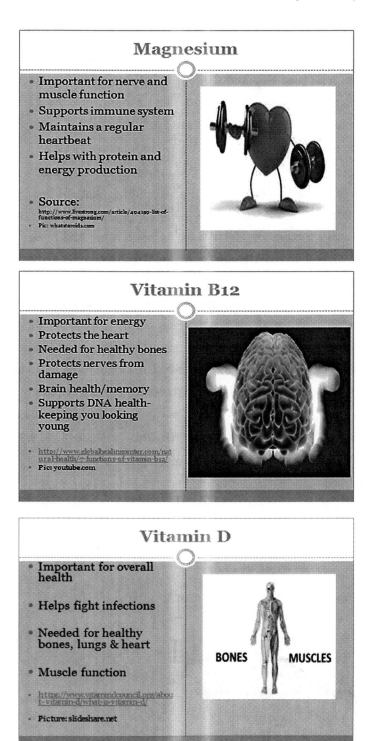

# Magnesium

- Important for nerve and muscle function
- Supports immune system
- Maintains a regular heartbeat
- Helps with protein and energy production

- Source:
  http://www.livestrong.com/article/494190-list-of-functions-of-magnesium/
- Pic: whatsteroids.com

# Vitamin B12

- Important for energy
- Protects the heart
- Needed for healthy bones
- Protects nerves from damage
- Brain health/memory
- Supports DNA health- keeping you looking young

- http://www.globalhealingcenter.com/natural-health/7-functions-of-vitamin-b12/
- Pic: youtube.com

# Vitamin D

- Important for overall health

- Helps fight infections

- Needed for healthy bones, lungs & heart

- Muscle function

- https://www.vitamindcouncil.org/about-vitamin-d/what-is-vitamin-d/

- Picture: slideshare.net

**BONES**    **MUSCLES**

It has been established in FMS and chronic pain that the body is in a constant state of stress thereby depleting the adrenal glands of some vital chemicals and hormones (especially cortisol). Explained in the slides below is the importance and affect some of the most important common nutritional deficiencies found in fibromyalgia.

As you read about all the possible treatments my hope and prayer is that you will recognize that when you treat the underlying cause instead of just pasting a Band-Aid across the symptoms, many of the issues can be FIXED with natural treatments. Food supplements with be discussed after natural supplements. Read with an open mind and remember this quote by Dr Pelligrino: "Today nutritional supplements are one of the most important treatments I recommend for fibromyalgia." I purposely did not list the recommended amount because everyone is different. However, you can purchase books or go online to find out the dosages. Please consult with physician, dietician or healthcare professional prior to starting. Lastly, I want to mention that I elaborated on magnesium because I wanted to stress the importance that many supplements may come in multiple forms and individual health considerations must be considered prior to taking them. To view the above slides in color, please visit my web site.

## INFORMATION ON SUPPLEMENTS

| Deficiency | Symptoms | Natural Supplements |
|---|---|---|
| Serotonin | Low blood sugar, increased pain, depression, fatigue | 5-HTP, St John's Wort, SAMe (pronounced Sammy) |
| Magnesium-see | Pain, muscle spasms, fatigue | Magnesium Maleate, Magnesium glycinate, works well with malic acid |

*Magnesium glycinate is the preferred form.

*Mg citrate-most popular-inexpensive-mild laxative, good for those with colon or bowel problems, unsuitable for those with loose BM

*Mg Taurate- best choice for those with heart issues, prevents arrhythmias, easily absorbed, no laxative effect

*Mag Maleate- fantastic choice for fatigue-because malic acid is a natural fruit acid and in most cells of the body, vital ingredient in enzymes that play key roles in ATP synthesis and energy production-absorbed well

*Mg Glycinate- one of the most bioavailable and absorbable forms of mg-least likely to cause diarrhea- safest for correct long term deficiency

*Mg chloride- easily absorbed- best form to take for detoxifying cells/tissues, aids kidney functions and boosts metabolism

*Mg Carbonate-popular and easily digested- good choice for those with acid reflux and indigestion-it contains ant-acid properties

*WORST forms of MAG: Mag oxide- most common form sold in drug stores-POOR absorption

*MG Sulfate- also called Epsom salt- fantastic for constipation, and soaking in a bath tub for sore muscles- can be unsafe d/t high potential of overdosing

*MG Glutamate & aspartate- dangerous components of aspartame-both can be neurotoxic

| | | |
|---|---|---|
| Amine ATP (energy molecules) | Fatigue, pain, muscle spasms | Magnesium, co-enzyme Q-10 |
| Vitamin B-12 | Weak immune system, numbness and tingling, fatigue | B-12 lozenges, sublingual B12, injections of B-12 |
| Low Growth Hormone (GH) | Weak immune system, fatigue increase in fibro fog, slowed metabolism | Colostrum, GH injections |
| Vitamin B-1 (thiamine) | Deficiency mimiks FMS symptoms | Thiamine |

| | | |
|---|---|---|
| Zinc | Associated with the number of tender points | Zinc |
| B-Complex Vitamin | Decreased energy, immunity, and nerve, and brain function | B-Complex vitamin |
| Adrenal hormone deficiency | Weakens immune system, inability to handle stress, increased anxiety | Colostrums, Vitamin C, Zinc, garlic, cinnamon, Echinacea |
| DHEA | Decrease in sex drive, dry eyes, skin, and hair, exhaustion, depression mood swings, problems with memory, loss of pubic hair, erectile dysfunction | Vitamon C, Panothenic Acid, Licorice root, Chromium |
| Anti-oxidants-supports overall cell & Immune function | Weak immune system, fatigue | Vitamins A & E, Lipoic Acid, Grapeseed extract |
| Vitamin D Deficiency | High blood pressure, depression, muscle weakness, bone pain | Sunshine, Vitamin D3 |
| MSM (methylsulfonylmethane) | ----------------------------- | Used for muscle and bone pain, rheumatoid arthritis, allergies and much more |
| **Supplements for treating Specific FM Symptoms** | | |
| Pain | Magnesium and malic acid, Glucosamine, chrondroitin, MSM, flaxseed oil, Tumeric (Helps a lot), Coenzyme Q10, Carnitine, 5-HTP, MSM | |
| Fatigue | Vitamin B-12, Ginko biloba, CoQ10, Magnesium and malic acid | |
| Poor Sleep | 5-HTP, Melatonin, Valerian Root, Lemon Balm, Passion flower | |
| Fibro Fog | Ginko biloba, Acetyl-L-carnitine | |
| Irritable Syndrome | Fiber supplements, Valerian root, Peppermint oil | |
| Depression | 5-HTP, St Johns Wort, Flaxseed oil, SAMe, | |
| Leaky Gut | Probiotics, multivitamin, Vitamin D & Zinc, Essential fish oils (especially Omega 3's) | |
| Anxiety | 5-HTP | |

(*https://www.womentowomen.com/general-womens-health-articles/a-natural-treatment-for-fibromyalgia-the-shine-approach/*)

# THE SHINE PROTOCOL

I came across some interesting information published by Dr. Jacob Teitelbaum, the world's famous fibro guru, in his book *The Fatigue and Fibromyalgia Solution,* which is a number one best seller on Amazon. In his introduction the doctor explained how he came down with CFS/FMS back in 1975 before there was a name designated to these conditions. He was attending med school, had to drop out because of his health, and became homeless. I am not quite sure how this happened, but he met multiple health practitioners who helped him get to the point where he could go back to medical school. He continued to research how to maximize his health, and others, for the past 30 years.

He has come up with a way to enhance and fill your energy tank. It's called the SHINE protocol. I will briefly explain what the doctor means by each of these. S stands for sleep. Dr. Teitelbaum explains how crucial sleep is. Getting 8-9 hours of sleep is ideal to replenish energy and heal. "H" stands for Hormones. Many CFS/FMS patients have hormone deficiencies that might need treatment. "I" stands for Infections. He suggests you get treatments for infections immediately when they occur. The lack of sleep ties to a weakened immune system and there can be underlying infections that contribute or even cause CFS/FM. "N" stands nutrition and he stresses that optimal nutritional supplements are critical. Many fibro and CFS patients suffer from nutritional deficiencies like B-12, magnesium, Vitamins D, C, and B which need to be supplemented at a dosage much higher than the average vitamin supplement provides. "E" stands for exercise as able. Dr. Teitelbaum says that after about 10 weeks on the first four steps that you will be able to slowly withstand an increase in ability to tolerate exercise. (Teitelbaum, 2013).

To learn more about the SHINE protocol, I recommend the book aforementioned in the above paragraph. There are also multiple web sites you can visit for more information: http://vitality101.com/, https://

www.womentowomen.com/general-womens-health-articles/a-natural-treatment-for-fibromyalgia-the-shine-approach/, https://secure.endfatigue.com/cfs-fibromyalgia/shine-protocol, http://www.preparemd.com/conditions/fatigue-shine-protocol-teitelbaum/. These web sites have an abundance of information and materials to educate yourself on natural supplements. Lastly, I'd like to mention that Dr Teitelbaum also does phone consultations with people worldwide. You can call 410-573-5389 and leave a voice mail, or e-mail Sarah at appointments@endfatigue.com.

## Natural Herbs/Spices

As with many natural supplements herbs, spices, or foods, you should be advised to check with your doctor to be sure there are no interactions between your meds and these natural items. One item in particular comes to mind when I mention this, and it is turmeric which has blood thinning properties. So if someone has bleeding tendencies or is already on a blood thinner, their doctor is likely going to advise them not to take turmeric.

Rather than try to list things out in paragraph form, I believe the best way to present this information is in chart format for quick reference. I have been collecting information for some time now. In addition, I have had others share information with me. However, be aware that there is so much more I need to learn, and so much more information out there that's available to be learned. Again, I re-iterate, educate yourself!

| Herb/Spice/Food | Health Benefit |
|---|---|
| St John's Wort-supplement | Anti-inflammatory, helps with pain |
| Boswellia- pregnant women should avoid this, may decrease the effect of other meds Healthline.com | Arthritis and Pain: Osteoarthritis, Rheumatoid Arthritis, Asthma, Breast Cancer, & Leukemia |
| Devil's Claw Arthritis.org | Relieves pain and inflammation for arthritis, lower back, knee and hip pain. May help lower uric acid levels in people with gout. |

| | |
|---|---|
| Boswellia- herb | FMS symptoms, back pain |
| Kava Kava-herb | Relaxes muscles, anxiety, insomnia |
| Cayenne- herb | Decreases pain signals |
| Ginger | Improves circulation, anti-inflammatory, pain relief, assists the immune system |
| Bromelain- (in pineapple juice) | Helps thin blood like Coumadin or aspirin, reduces pain and inflammation |
| Cat's Claw-a fungicide *could interfere with other meds | Decreases inflammation, improves the immune system |
| Chlorella | Decreases pain |
| Willow Bark Tea –this is what aspirin is made from | Reduces pain, without the side effect of upset stomach like aspirin |
| Tumeric-herb-has blood thinning properties | Anti-inflammatory=decreasing pain |
| Lavender- herb | Anti-inflammatory=pain relief and decreased swelling, relaxing scent helps to sleep and overall many FMS symptoms |
| Source for above info: healthheal.info | |
| Licorice Root- herb  Side effects: swelling, high blood pressure, low potassium, chronic fatigue, don't take longer than 4 weeks | Anti-inflammatory, heartburn, female reproductive issues, leaky gut, adrenal fatigue, helps immune system, PMS |
| Cinnamon | Anti-inflammatory, protects the heart, improves mental alertness, helps circulation, arthritis and muscle pain |
| Ginger | Helps with nausea, immune system, and digestion, is also an anti-viral, helps osteoarthritis |
| Resource: draxe.com & naturalnews.com | |
| Hibiscus Tea- has a sour taste like cranberry | Helps lower blood pressure and cholesterol, aids with digestive, immune and inflammation, liver health, weight loss, speeds metabolism, lots of vitamin C helps anxiety, anti-cancer properties, PMS, promotes skin health |
| L-Glutamine | Helps heal intestinal lining |
| Probiotics | Promotes good intestinal bacteria |
| Oregano Oil | Rich in anti-oxidants, helps strengthen immune system, helps balance good and bad intestinal bacteria |

| Purified water with Organic Apple Cider Vinegar (ACV) | ACV is loaded with enzymes that promote good intestinal bacteria, strengthens immune system |
|---|---|
| Iodine | Supports the immune system, defends against microorganisms, helps thyroid health |
| Fresh Lemon Water<br><br><br><br><br>Source: healthylifebox | *In the morning on an empty stomach lemon will flush out toxins<br><br>*Anti-inflammatory properties-will help respiratory & tonsil infections, & sore throats<br><br>*The citric acid aids digestion<br><br>*Contains pectin which suppresses cravings & hunger- helps with weight loss<br><br>*Stimulates the liver to release toxins, thus helping to clean the liver |

## FIBRO FOODS

Well, here's a section you may or may not be looking forward to. We are what we eat! It wasn't until I admitted to myself that I was ignoring this important aspect of caring for my illness, that I realized how critical the foods I was eating was contributing to how bad I felt. I assure you, along with many other credible references, that nutrition plays a huge role in fibro. While it's true that medications may help treat the symptoms of fibro, it does not fix an underlying problem that exists with production of important amino acids and nutrition. Dietary intake and supplements are where we will get the much needed building blocks to fix what is broken.

According to the National Fibromyalgia Research Association, patients with fibro are often urged to limit sugar, caffeine, and alcohol because they irritate muscles and stress our system. Thus, proper nutrition can be helpful in thwarting stress, helping to dispose of toxins, and restoring nutrition. Again, please consult with your family doctor, nutritional specialist, or functional medicine doctor before you start any new nutritional program because as previously mentioned there can be dangerous side effects if certain supplements or therapies are mixed with certain medications.

I want to ensure I mention the concept of juicing prior to listing healthy foods and their benefits. I own a nutra-bullet (for nutrition extraction) but do not use it as often as I should. However, after writing this book and equipping myself with so much information, I have made a vow to do better. According to nutri-bullet.com, extraction is better than juicing or blending because it breaks down the cell walls of fruits and vegetables and releases vitamins and minerals which give you the highest amount of nutrition possible.

If you relate that back to the leaky gut problem and nutrition deficit many of us suffer, it will make sense to you as to why we need to make nutrition as readily available and highly absorbable as possible. I love the words I read in an article that said ""heal-thy" self. This process will indeed help lead us to a path of better nutrition. If you visit nutria-bullet.com and scroll to the bottom of the page, you will find some healthy recipes.

As promised, I have some information on how you can help your leaky gut syndrome. As a quick review I want to remind you how leaky gut develops. It is multifactorial but the main causes include: overuse of antibiotics, gluten, poor diet, chronic stress, and an imbalance of good and bad bacteria in your gut.

It's vital that you stay away from grains and gluten containing wheat while trying to heal your leaky gut. Regular pasteurized cow's milk can also cause a leaky gut, so almond or coconut milk is recommended. Stay away from refined sugar which feeds the yeast and causes overgrowth of it. This was previously mentioned, but worth mentioning again because it's vital because sugar produces toxins that damage the cells of the gut.

Dr Josh Axe has a new book out titled, *Eat Dirt* which I have purchased. In it he thoroughly describes and explains leaky gut and a program to follow to help heal your leaky gut. Much of it is making simple changes like quit eating out of Teflon coated pans, because when heated to a certain degree, it releases a chemical damaging to the body. Also, as a society we are becoming too clean. For example, using no wash hand sanitizer. This can actually remove the good basteria living on our skin. Additionally, many of the perfumes and cleaning items we use are full of harmful chemicals.

For the sake of time, I am going to use DR Axe's four steps found at http://draxe.com/4-steps-to-heal-leaky-gut-and-autoimmune-disease/, to help you get a jump start with leaky gut syndrome. The four steps are: 1.) Remove, 2.) Replace, 3.) Repair, 4.) Rebalance. Additionally, omega 3 fatty acids have anti-inflammatory properties that fights the auto immune response prompted by the leaky gut syndrome. See chart below for more information.

| Remove damaging foods and factors | Replace with healing foods | Repair with certain supplements | Rebalance with Probiotics |
|---|---|---|---|
| Gluten<br>Dairy<br>Refined sugars<br>Foods you are allergic to<br>As much stress as possible<br>Wheat<br>Grains<br>Soda pop<br>Unbalanced diet | *Bone broth:contains collagen and amino acids that heal cells<br>*Fermented veggies such as sauerkraut.<br>*Coconut foods are esp good for the gut. (coconut Kefir-has probiotics)<br>*Sprouted seeds help the growth of good bacteria in the gut. (Examples: chia, flax, and hemp seeds | ***Probiotics-most important due to helping restock good bacteria and crowd out the bad.<br>*L-Glutamine: Heals and protects<br>*Licorice root: balances cortisol and helps acid production in stomach<br>* Quercetin: helps seal the gut | ** Probiotic capsules<br>Probiotic Foods:<br>-Yogurt with live and active cultures<br>-Unpasteurized sauerkraut,<br>- Miso Soup<br>- Soft Cheeses<br>- Kefir: a drink<br>- Sourdough Bread<br>-Sour pickles |

Once more, there are a multitude of foods that could be mentioned within this section. If you will refer to the information below, I will share my data I have collected along my journey. If you wish to know more, you can refer to the nutritional resources I will provide at the end of the chapter, or you can simply google "fibro foods" or anti-inflammatory foods" and you will get thousands of sources.

    a.) Anti-oxidants: Fresh organic fruits and veggies, Pecans, walnuts, and hazelnuts, grapeseed oil, Purple, Red, and Blue Grapes, blueberries, red berries, dark green veggies, sweet potatoes, orange vegetables, tea- especially green tea, whole grains, beans, fish, red wine, cranberries (Elaine Magee, MPH, RD, the "Recipe Doctor" for WebMD)

    b.) Foods for pain relief:

1. Ginger: anti-inflammatory, muscle and joint pain

2. Olive Oil: contains ingredients similar to ibuprofen

3. Salmon: contains Omega 3's, reduces joint pain and inflammation

4. Red Grapes: contains resveratrol-anti-inflammatory

5. Thyme: contains dexamethasone which reduces pain perception

6. Fish Oil: contains chemicals to block inflammation

7. Tart Cherries: said to work better that aspirin, works for arthritis, gout, and inflammation

8. Apple cider vinegar: reduces inflammation

9. Coconut oil: anti-inflammatory, good for joint and back pain

10. Onions and garlic: reduces inflammation

11. Chia seeds: good also as an anti-oxidant and a great source of Omega 3 fatty acids

12. Orange and red vegetables: decreases inflammation

13. Dark Green Leafy Vegetables: fights inflammation

14. Chile Peppers: contains capsaicin which blocks pain signals

15. Cherries: contains anthocyanins which are anti-inflammatories, also thought to help increase muscle strength (http://www.bodyand-soul.com.au/nutrition/nutrition+tips/five+foods+that+fight+pain,17421)

| Healing Herbal Teas | Benefits |
|---|---|
| Green Tea | Protects from aging, boosts metabolism=weight loss, fights cancer, heart disease |
| Chamomile | Promotes sleep, boosts immune system, helps with anxiety & Depression |
| Mint | Helps with stress and anxiety, promotes sleep, natural appetite suppressant, helps with bloating and gas, helps balance hormones, soothes muscles |
| Thyme | Fights bacteria and fungi, strong anti-inflammatory, healthy for your heart |
| Lemon Verbena | Helps with digestion, calms the nervous system, breaks down fat |
| Nettle | Reduces leg cramps, great source of iron and calcium, helps urinary system, counters arthritis, decreases blood sugar and blood pressure |
| Ginger | Relieves stress, anxiety, helps nausea, digestion, and blood circulation, helps immune system, clears sinuses, helps congestion |

I have spoke a lot about inflammation which can mean infection which often leads to pain, but it can mean other things. Inflammatory processes are the body's attempt to protect itself, rid the body of damaged cells, harmful invaders, and aid in healing. It is indeed a part of the body's immune response. So inflammation is not always a bad thing, especially when dealing with an acute infection. However, when chronic illness strikes, it's the prolonged inflammatory process that causes the body to turn upon itself. So for those of us with chronic illness there are multiple foods we can chose to eat to help ourselves. Here is a list of some:

| Basil | Black pepper | Cloves | Cayenne pepper | Chives | Cilantro |
|---|---|---|---|---|---|
| Oregano | Nutmeg | Parsley | Rosemary | Tumeric | alfalfa |
| Almonds | Almond butter | Artichokes | Avocado | Bee pollen | Brussel sprouts |
| Buckwheat | Cabbage | Caraway seeds | Cauliflower | Celery | Fresh coconut |
| Cucumbers | Cumin seeds | Egg plant | Fennel seeds | Figs | Kale |
| Leeks | Fresh lemon | Lentils | lettuce | Fresh limes | Mustard greens |
| zucchini | yam | White or red radishes | Seaweed | pumpkin | onions |
| Fresh peas | Mustard greens | Fresh limes | spinach | squash | Sweet potatoes |
| Sesame seeds | rutabaga | Fresh red beets | parsnips | Bok choy | ~~tomatoes~~ |
| onion | spelt | almonds | Apple cider vinegar | apricots | asparagus |
| avocado | blueberries | raspberries | blackberries | beans | broccoli |
| Cantaloupe | Carrots | Cinnamon | Curry Powder | Dark chocolate | Eggs |
| Extra Virgin Olive Oil | Flaxseed | Garlic | Grapefruit | Ginger | Kiwi |
| kelp | Oats | Oranges | Papaya | Pineapple | Quinoa |
| http://bembu.com/quinoa-benefits | | | | | |

Since we have talked about the many foods you should eat, I'd like to mention foods now that those with fibromyalgia or chronic pain should avoid. MSG, or monosodium glutamate, and sodium nitrate are food additives and also a neurotransmitter that excites and possibly stimulates pain receptors. Stevia is the recommended sweetener for those of us with chronic pain. You have heard all the way through that you should limit sugar, but why? When we eat sugar, our insulin rises to allow sugar to be used; and an elevated insulin level can intensify pain. Here are a few more things to remember:

1. Try to avoid nightshade vegetables which are tomatoes, potatoes, & eggplant.

2. Avoid aspartame which is a chemical that increases one's sensitivity to pain. Aspartame in particular is known to trigger fibromyalgia symptoms Aspartame is often found in diet sodas, and sugar free items. Aspartame is a chemical that the body converts to formaldehyde.

3. Avoid junk food which may lead to weight gain, the development of harmful eating habits, as well as cause problems with sleeping, muscle irritation, and weaken the immune system.

   (http://articles.mercola.com/sites/articles/archive/2010/01/19/foods-that-chronic-pain-sufferers-need-to-avoid.aspx)

4. Try to avoid gluten which is found in wheat, rye, and barley items. Gluten fuels inflammation throughout your entire body which produces migraines, constipation, diarrhea, acid reflux, digestive issues, fatigue, and mental function. (http://www.prohealth.com/library/showarticle.cfm?libid=18639, http://articles.mercola.com/sites/articles/archive/2010/01/19/foods-that-chronic-pain-sufferers-need-to-avoid.aspx).

I thought it would be nice to share a few recipes collected from my fibro Facebook support group for those of you who are looking for a healthy way to get started. The first recipe comes from Tammy Holsman who says: I use kefir milk in a smoothie. About 3/4 cup of kefir to 1/2 can of v8 fusion juice add some strawberries and blueberries and ice with one pkg of carnation breakfast vanilla powder blend; great smoothie for energy vitamin and protein.

Here is another recipe from another member. Lenora Ziobro says she uses Green tea with ginger, turmeric, Cheyenne pepper, camomile, Basil, rosemary, nutmeg, cinnamon and honey. I also have smoothies in the morning that have fruit including pineapple and blueberries among others, spinach, ginger, nutmeg, and most important, coconut oil.

In concluding the discussion regarding food, the best kinds of food come from nature; fresh fruits and vegetables. More specifically the deepest color fruits and vegetables contain the most nutrients. Additionally, staying away from junk foods, diet foods, and gluten will likely lessen your intake of chemicals and sugar that could stimulate pain.

## HOMEOPATHY & CAT

Homeopathic medicine and physicians practice under the belief that the body has the ability to heal itself. Unfortunately it is not included in traditional medical training in the US or Great Britain (www.webmd.com/balance/guide/hemeopathy-topic-overview). Homeopathic physicians use mostly all natural treatments for their patients and treat the patients holistically (mind, body, and spirit). If medication is needed they will use it but in very diluted ways. Homeopathic treatments are less expensive than medicine, minimal side effects, thus making them safe.

I came across a study regarding the flu and homeopathic treatments. Results showed that those treated naturally recovered 48 hours sooner than those who took medication. There are multiple conditions that can be treated homeopathically " including infections, circulatory problems, respiratory problems, heart disease, depression and nervous disorders, migraine headaches, allergies, arthritis, and diabetes" (http://medical-dictionary.thefreedictionary.com/homeopathic+medicine). Some examples of homeopathic medicine are as follows:

1. Allium cepa (onion): treats the common cold or hay fever
2. Arnica (mountain daisy): used for pain. I have used the gel form and it does help.

3. Chamomile: beneficial for sleep, infants who are teething or have colic

4. Ignatia (St. Ignatius bean): for grief, anxiety, and depression

5. Nux vomica (poison nut): treats overeating and commonly used for drug and alcohol addictions

6. Rhus tox (poison ivy): used for sprains and strains **(https://www.ho-meopathic.com/Articles/Introduction_to_Homeopathy/Ten_Common_Ho-meopathic_Medicines.html)**

7. Yoder apple cider vinegar or ACV: made by the Amish and contains 14 herbs and spices as well as fermented apple cider vinegar; used for arthritis, digestion, pain, circulation, anxiety, benefits the immune system, and much more. Additional uses can be found at: **http://www.moderndaydads.com/daily-photo-23/. (http://www.yoders-goodhealthrecipe.com/index.html)**

Complimentary Alternative Medicine (CAT) is a branch of medical treatment where no medications or surgery is included. Some of the CAT's are making a big comeback such as yoga, acupuncture, and aroma therapy. For those with fibromyalgia or who suffer from chronic pain, it has been my experience that these types of therapy are an extremely important part of therapy in treating pain. I am going to include some techniques you will have heard of, and perhaps some you have not heard of.

The first therapy I would like to start with is called "Floating." Flotation therapy has been studied both in the US and Sweden and results show that it reduces pain, stress, blood pressure, but increases blood flow, which is beneficial. These floatation tanks include approximately 10 inches of water loaded with between 1,000- 2,000 pounds of Epsom salt which contains magnesium that is absorbed readily through our skin.

The "Floating" concept provides zero gravity which is the only place on earth you can experience this. I had to laugh as I came across an article titled "Adult size wombs are taking over the meditation world." I never knew this existed until I heard of it within my fibromyalgia FB support group. I was immediately intrigued and searched for a place in my area I could try it. After finding one in Midland Michigan, I called mi Float, then my friend and I went and floated for an hour. The process I followed was showering and washing my hair before and after the float. They provide ear plugs so the salt water doesn't get in your ears. A small air filled neck pillow is also provided.

I had the choice as to whether I wanted meditation music playing; I could control the volume, and even have the lights on if I wanted. You get into the pod with no clothes on because I was told clothes could contaminate the pod. The next hour was absolutely heavenly. I listened to relaxing music and tried to turn my brain off for the first 15 minutes or so. However, after that I felt myself more relaxed than ever before in my life. My friend said that was the most awesome and relaxing thing she had ever done. Both of us agreed it was much better than having a massage.

I would like to provide a picture as an example of what a float pod looks like, compliments of mi Float in Midland Michigan and there web site is as follows: http://www.mifloatmidland.com/

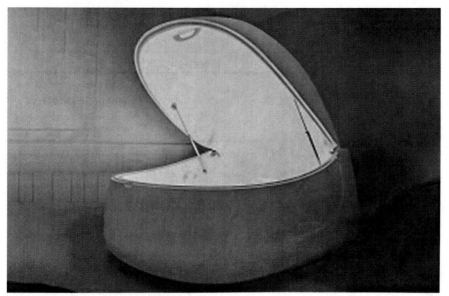

Soaking in Epsom salt can be done at home as well. Epsom salt provides many benefits to the mind, body and spirit by helping you sleep better, look better, have more energy, reduce adrenaline effects thus feel relaxed, improve thinking and concentration, nerve function, muscle cramps, pain and function, relieve pain in general, relieve constipation, and help the body rid toxins. For stress relief it is recommended you take an Epsom salt bath three times a week and add 2 cups of Epsom salt to your hot bath and soak for at least 12 minutes. There are multiple other uses for Epsom salt that I had never heard of that benefit your health, but can also be used outdoors for a green lawn and pesticide. Here are but a few more benefits we can use Epsom salt for: athlete's foot, removes splinters, treats toenail fungus, sprains and bruises, helps gout pain, to exfoliate skin, and eliminates foot odor. (https://www.seasalt. com/salt-101/epsom-salt-uses-benefits). http://www.hopefloatsusa.com/en/flo-tation-therapy/about/

There are so many alternative therapies and I would like to tell you every single one I have collected information on. However, that is not realistic. I will mention some that you may be familiar with and some you may not have heard of. Again, please consult with your doctor to make sure there is no medical contraindication for you to try the therapy

| Therapy | Additional info |
| --- | --- |
| Magnet therapy | The use of energy and electrical current to stimulate cells and enhance physical and emotional health. Those with pacemakers should NOT do this. |
| Aroma therapy/Essential Oil Therapy: When you smell it's believed to stimulate the parts of your brain that can influence physical, mental and emotional health. | Used to help pain, mood improvement, relaxation, reduces anxiety, depression, and stress. Example: orange blossom=calming<br><br>It can be inhaled through a diffuser, used directly on skin, and consumed- although consumption should be handled by professionals only- not all oils can be ingested. |

| | |
|---|---|
| Humor therapy | Laughter is a natural pain killer via releasing endorphins, helps lose weight, decreases stress, reduces heart disease (ebjchechcastro). |
| Pet therapy | Helps relieve symptoms of fibro |
| Music Therapy<br>*Facebook page: Fibromyalgia Support* | Relaxation, decreases pain, helps people cope with physical, spiritual, &psychological pain. Anxiety & depression, improves sleep |
| Emu oil | Pain relief |
| Acupuncture<br>Traditional Chinese treatment for pain | Insertion of needles placed strategically to stimulate nerves, muscles, and connective tissue, which is thought to increase blood flow and release body's natural pain killers (mayoclinic.org). |
| Accupressure | Uses the same principle as acupuncture-except with the use of gentle to firm pressure with fingers. Helps to detoxify the body, better sex, back pain, emotional pain. |
| Chiropractic care | To help with spinal alignment and pain |
| Reflexology | Using impulses to help healthy circulation of cerebro-spinal fluid through the brain and spinal cord-helping to relieve pain |
| Craniosacral therapy | Using impulses to help healthy circulation of cerebro-spinal fluid through the brain and spinal cord-helping to relieve pain |
| Reiki<br>Holistic Japanese Therapy | Uses a light feather touch to encourage health of the whole body |
| Aromatherapy | Uses specific smells to help relax |
| Hypnosis | Helps with: Phobias, fears, PTSD, and anxiety. Promotes sleep, helps with grief and depression |
| Meditation<br>- a form of relaxation that uses concentrated focusing on breathing and clearing your mind<br>Usually involves the mind and body | Helps muscle relaxation, promotes oxygen flow which helps healing, helps produce melanin (needed for deep sleep), decreases depression and anxiety, minimizes migraines |

| | |
|---|---|
| Yoga<br>There are multiple types of yoga<br>Low impact- stretching<br>Hatha-focuses on specific poses and actions | Teaches people how to control breathing, relaxes muscles, enhances mobility, and helps reduce stress |
| Reflexology:<br>Application of pressure to certain areas on hands, feet, or ears (mayoclinic.org) | May reduce pain, depression, anxiety, help sleep<br>If you Google reflexology-you will see that our whole body is mapped out on the hands and feet. |
| Trigger point therapy | Relieves referred pain associated with trigger points- injections, massage, physical therapy |
| Massage Therapy | Lessens pain via releasing endorphins, migraines, increases muscle circulation which aids in detoxifying and delivering nutrients, relaxes muscles, and improves joint mobility |
| Myofascial Release-tender knots: Inflammation of soft tissue or connective tissue covering muscles- (Clevelandclinic.org) | Gentle pressure applied to myofascial connective tissue (mayoclinic.org) |
| Aerobics/water aerobics:<br>Regular aerobics is often too rigorous- so water aerobics is often a better alternative | Mobility and gaining strength is important to keep muscles from wasting away. |
| Swimming | Allows less pressure and pain on joints, improves mobility and flexibility, decreases overall pain and increases overall quality of life. |

*Massage envy.com*

I'd like to elaborate on a couple therapies mentioned above. The first one is the essential oil therapy. There is a recipe I came across online called a Morphine Bomb Recipe created by Carla Green. The recipe calls for: 5 drops of Copaiba, Idaho Balsam Fir, and Frankincense placed in a vegetable capsule. This recipe provides pain relief for migraines, arthritis, fibro, back injuries and other pain. Copaiba oil contains highest amounts of Beta-caryophyllene, which is found in marijuana, blocking pain signals, thereby decreasing inflammation.

Through Young Living Oils there's a sleepy cream which calls for ¾ cup organic coconut oil, 8 drops of lavender, peace and calming, and valor. There is also a bath salt for detoxification which consists of 3 drops of lemon and peppermint oil and ½ cup of Epsom salt, then soak for 30 minutes. Lastly a pain cream recipe consists of ¾ cup of organic coconut oil, 8 drops of valor, Pan away, Peppermint, and lemongrass. This combination should be whipped and stored in a dark jar.

In conclusion, there are multiple ways for people with fibromyalgia or chronic pain to help themselves with traditional, functional medicine, or a combination of both. I want to testify to some of the complimentary alternative methods and their effectiveness. Floating, meditation, deep breathing, water therapy, aroma therapy, essential oils, emu oil, humor therapy, and pet therapy have been effective for me. The floating has been, by far, the most effective for my muscle soreness and overall pain relief as well as reaching a state of relaxation.

## RESOURCES:

1. American Kratom Association: Americankratomassociation.org

2. The Kratom User's Guide: www.sagewisdom.org/kratomguide.html

3. Fibromyalgia: What to eat, what not to eat: http://www.everyday-health.com/fibromyalgia/fibromyalgia/what-to-eat-what-not-to-eat.aspx

4. Foods that Help, Foods that Hurt: http://www.everydayhealth.com/fibromyalgia-pictures/eat-well-to-help-fibromyalgia.aspx

5. Fibro Nutrition; Vitamins and minerals are essential: http://www.fibromyalgiahope.com/fibromyalgia-nutrition.html

6. Fibro Nutrition and Diet Therapy: http://www.holistic-online.com/Remedies/cfs/fib_nutrition.htm

7. Foods that fight inflammation: http://www.health.harvard.edu/staying-healthy/foods-that-fight-inflammation

8. Top 15 anti-inflammatory foods: http://draxe.com/anti-inflammatory-foods/

9. Anti-inflammatory Diet: http://www.drweil.com/drw/u/ART02012/anti-inflammatory-diet

10. Healthy Recipes and Tips: http://www.epicurious.com/archive/healthy

# CHAPTER 6

---

# THE LATEST AND GREATEST

*Somewhere something incredible*
*is waiting to be known*

*~Unknown*

Many of you have been suffering from FMS before anyone was willing to admit that it even existed. Thankfully, there have been some advances in research and the illness even has its own diagnostic code and is recognized as an official illness. So even though it may not feel like it, fibromyalgia has come a long way. Even Social Security Disability has made some revisions in the way it acknowledges and goes through the evaluation process as to whether approve or not approve disability. I will cover tips and tricks that I have learned about the disability process in Chapter 7. However, in this chapter I want to talk about some of the cutting edge issues and research that are bringing attention and helping to legitimize fibromyalgia as real.

## FIBRO BLOOD TEST

As I was researching fibro I was fortunate enough to come across information regarding a new blood test. As many of you know, currently fibro is being treated as a diagnosis of exclusion. This means that multiple conditions must be ruled out before fibro can be ruled in and that there are really NO diagnostic tests for FMS. However, I am extremely excited to share some developing information with you. I have had the honor and opportunity to speak with and interview Dr. Bruce Gillis who is an internal medicine specialist, researcher, and CEO of Epigenics located in Santa Monica, California. His hospital affiliation is with Cedars-Sinai Medical Center in Los Angeles, CA.

Originally a fibromyalgia skeptic, he explained the test to me like this: The blood test FM/a includes isolating white blood cells (WBC) and then stimulating them within a lab setting to determine whether they fail to have the capacity to provide vital proteins called cytokines and chemokines. In documented studies he stated that Fibromyalgia patients have decreased amounts of proteins which proves there is a dysfunction of their immune systems. This is not the same thing as an autoimmune disease where the body actually attacks itself because it does not recognize itself. "It is absolutely not an autoimmune disease," stated Dr. Gillis during my phone interview on 10/20/15.

Dr. Gillis stated his objective is to legitimize the diagnosis of fibromyalgia as an actual disease and to set objective criteria that patients can be evaluated by. He also shared with me that there is a unique set of biomarkers specific to FM. The sensitivity of this test is 93%. Of course no test or anything in medicine is 100%.

Currently, fibro is a rule out condition meaning that when a patient comes in and the doctors are uncertain as to what is wrong with the patients, then a myriad of labs and diagnostic testing is ordered to rule out any other disease or condition. The diagnostic process for FMS is said to take between three to five years and cost between \$4,900-\$9,300 per year. This translates to a needless waste of years and thousands of dollars. In contrast, the the FM/a blood test is a "Rule-in" test.

Dr. Gillis hopes to further conduct studies to see if there is a genetic component by extracting and studying their RNA. However, more research requires more money. In order to raise more research money, the test needs to be utilized by the medical community. Unfortunately, practitioners are not lining up to support this test for many reasons. First, if they order the test and get a positive diagnosis of fibro then they do not need to have the patient come back for repeated visits, labs and diagnostics. Thus, they lose income. Drug companies have much to lose because if FM is declared a disorder of the immune system, then medications can be more targeted and focused in on Fibromyalgia as opposed to a patient going through trial and error for many years to simply put a Band-Aid on their symptoms. Additionally, there are a multitude of alternative and homeopathic remedies that work, as evidenced a multitude of statements made by Fibro sufferers- see below for patient statements. Therefore those drug companies have much to lose in the way of income as well.

There are, as always, a few skeptics out there who are declaring that Dr. Gillis' study doesn't have a large enough sample to support his results. I have also found out that there was a neurologist in Germany who fought to have Dr. Gillis' study from being published because it would contradict her studies and theories she has been working on for years now. Dr. Gillis fought back with a rebuttal and won the rights to publish his article.

I asked Dr. Gillis about another one of his critics; especially Dr. Wolfe who calls this junk science. Dr. Wolfe says Dr. Gillis' research and test studies are bad because the sample sizes and amount of studies are extremely limited. However, given the chance to refute or ask questions during the annual convention of the American College of Rheumatology,

Dr. Wolfe admitted he had been paid hundreds of thousands of dollars by Pfizer, a drug company that sells billions of dollars of Lyrica which has no immune system benefits.

Furthermore, he told me for every 100 doctors there are approximately 90 who are either skeptics or do not believe in fibromyalgia despite the fact that FM is recognized as a diagnosable condition by the United States National Institute of Health and The American College Of Rheumatology.

Upon investigating how the test works, it's fairly simple and I will explain the steps below. I went through all the steps and was going to have the test performed on myself, but found out I would have to be off my steroids for five days. That is impossible for me as I suffer from severe adrenal insufficiency and if I stop taking steroids, my Cleveland clinic physician said I would end up in the hospital in an adrenal crisis. The other criteria that would exclude a patient on anti-cancer and anti-rejection medications that patients have to take after an organ transplant.

The cost of the test at the time I spoke to Dr. Gillis was $794, which includes the Fed-Ex handling fees. I am informed that the test is covered 100% by Medicare, and some other insurance companies are starting to cover the test as well. It would be advisable to call your insurance company if you want to know if your specific company will cover the test. I would also suggest calling the billing number on the epigenetics website. If you or your health care professionals have questions or need information about the blood test, the web site is: https://thefibromyalgiatest.com/

So how does the test work? Here are the steps:

1.) Speak to your doctor so you can get an order for it. Suggestion: make a copy of what the blood test is from the healthcare professional site and be prepared to give it to your doctor. When I went in to see my new rheumatologist, who is the best in our area, she had not heard of the test. She was, however, interested and open to accepting the information I had for her. She also agreed to order the test, and did.

Here are the steps:

1. Have the physician fax the completed form to the number provided directly on the form.

2. The company will contact you with financial information.

3. If all is well, they will have the supplies sent to you via Fed-Ex and you will go to any lab to get the blood drawn.

4. Then you will follow mailing instructions-and sent it back to the lab via Fed-Ex.

5. You will have your results within a week.

See below for the pertinent web sites:

Fibromyalgia Blood test:

1. General information: http://nationalpainreport.com/new-fibromyalgia-blood-test-is-99-accurate-8821072.html

2. Questions and Answers about the blood test for patients: https://thefibromyalgiatest.com/?page_id=1402

3. Information for Healthcare Professionals. If your doctor has never heard of the test-or would like more information, here is a link: https://thefibromyalgiatest.com/?page_id=1416

4. Physicians Authorization & Order Form: Plus a Fax Number to send it to https://thefibromyalgiatest.com/?page_id=1418

5. Billing telephone number: 1-877-270-4480

## DNA TESTING

Another piece of information I'd like to pass along has to do with DNA testing to determine adverse reactions to medication. According to kvue. com this testing is covered by 100% by Medicare. Reportedly 136 billion dollars was spent on adverse drug reactions in the year 2013. Although we are all human, our DNA differs from one individual to the next. We are all chemically a bit different is an easier way to explain it. Genetic testing can arm doctors with a defense to prevent these life threatening reactions.

The test is very easy and starts with just a swab on the insides of both the patient's cheeks which can give doctors vital information as to how their system will react with certain medications. I only wish I would have known this prior to taking the Z-pack I was prescribed for my bronchitis. I suffered a severe allergic reaction that almost ended my life. Ever since then, my health has snowballed downhill and I firmly believe that is when my body turned on itself in every way possible. So I developed fibromyalgia, rheumatoid arthritis, adrenal insufficiency among many other health problems. I went from an active type A personality working 12 hour shifts as a nurse and nursing instructor, to someone who spent every other month in the hospital for 2-3 weeks at a time. I eventually lost my career due to inability to function, and then reluctantly applied for disability and was approved.

Back to the DNA testing information regarding adverse med reactions; Dr. Lichtenhan says this test is a tool and can offer not only genetic traits but ways to modify treatments. An example used is a patient that comes in and says that a pain med is not working effectively to control the pain. This test can actually help the doctor dissect how the body metabolizes the drug. The goal is to develop a "super pill" that can be made especially for your body type so your body will process it and the pill will be effective for you.

Unfortunately, genetic testing is expensive, but as previously mentioned Medicare has agreed to pay for the test, and other insurance companies are following suit. If you give it serious thought, the cost of genetic testing is almost positively cheaper than having to treat a patient with medications for a lifelong health problem, such as the multiple health problems I have developed. So in conclusion, genetic testing can be used to not only help reduce and prevent adverse medication reactions, but also to help prevent health problems because reactions to meds can be toxic and life threatening.

## PERSONAL EXPERIENCE WITH FUNCTIONAL MEDICINE DOCTOR: DR. ROGER MURPHREE

Moving on, I'd like to now expand on some exciting information I have learned about treating FMS and chronic illness naturally. I am currently working with Dr. Rodger Murphree. Dr. Murphree has been treating FM for approximately 20 years and has emphatically told me that you do not have to accept the statement given to many fibro patients that "you'll just have to learn to live with this." In fact, he told me to communicate with all of you folks reading this book that you should reject that notion because it simply is not true.

Prior to going any further, I do want to emphasize that every FM case is different because we are all individuals. Additionally, each of us has different co-morbid conditions to deal with. This information must be kept in the back of your mind as you read the information I am going to share.

So how did I come across Dr Murphree? As I was investigating and learning about fibro during my journey to write this book as well as educate myself, Dr. Murphree's name kept popping up everywhere I looked. He is located in Birmingham Alabama, so I was intrigued as to how the process would work since I live in Michigan. However, his web site www.yourfibrodoctor.com says that he helps people all over the world.

I was also very inspired by the statement "I am on a mission to help you feel better and get your life back again" which is located on his home web page. The words "YOU AREN'T CRAZY" were also reassuring and comforting, because at times I really did feel like I was losing my mind. Furthermore, I was impressed by the fact that his web site offered free live webinars every Tuesday, a free download regarding three keys you must know to beat and treat your fibromyalgia, and multiple other free resources, listen to past teleconferences, sign up for free newsletter and much more. He seemed to really care about helping people.

I must communicate that prior to calling Dr. Murphree, my health was in very bad shape. I was homebound and spent many days in bed. Physical therapy had even discharged me because I could not participate. I felt like I was at the end of my rope and that this was my last hope for any kind of a life. I was merely existing and felt as if life was passing me by.

Prior to speaking with Dr. Murphree on the phone, I filled out a comprehensive health history form and sent it via e-mail. My initial consult with Dr. Murphree was $129.00, but worth every penny. After our discussion, he told me that there was no doubt in his mind he could not only help me, but also could give me a better quality of life, and get me to a better state of health. However, I have multiple complicating factors. I have an extensive health history, with many other diagnoses besides FM. In the words of Dr. Murphree, which I will never forget, "You are lucky to be alive."

So during my consultation we reviewed my history and he asked me multiple questions starting with my sleeping pattern, which was basically non-existent. After quite a lengthy conversation we spoke about a program that was specific for me as an individual. Yes, it was expensive but as I prayed about it afterward, my prayer was answered this way: "You cannot put a price on your health." So I proceeded forward with confidence that I was not in a hopeless situation.

Dr. Murphree started with helping me work on getting better sleep. His comment echoed what my medical internist told me, "If you don't get sleep, you won't get well." Sleep is essential for multiple reasons as mentioned in chapter 1; however in relationship to dietary reasons, serotonin reduces overeating and sugar cravings. Something I did not know about insufficient sleep is that our body will store fat instead of burning it. (Dr. Murphree, 2014)

Prior to starting my program, Dr. Murphree ordered a panel of labs as well as food allergies. No physician had ever tested me for food allergies. The results were astounding. I have 26 food allergies. I didn't know I had any food allergies at all. I am sure they contributed greatly to my leaky gut which no doubt I have because I exhibit all the signs and symptoms.

As time went on we had to tweak a few of the supplements to help me sleep. I will list the supplements I take and their functions at the end of this chapter. We spoke on the phone every week to begin with because he wanted to keep close tabs and make sure we were making forward progress. Being a nurse, I have dealt with hundreds of doctors over the years and I know when one cares as opposed to not. I was very impressed with the compassion and caring demeanor that Dr. Murphree displayed and knew I had made the right decision to work with him.

After I started sleeping a bit better, we moved forward and started working on dietary changes. I started on an elimination diet, which means I eliminated the foods I was allergic to which included gluten, and many other things. I also eliminated all concentrated sources of sugars, oils, and butter. Other things I eliminated were all dairy, sodas, and decreasing my caffeine intake.

The elimination of sugar is vital because it feeds the yeast in our intestines. In fact, it's the yeast that causes us to crave sugars. So we must starve the yeast. Did you know that too much sugar can suppress the immune system, speed the aging process, and contribute to depression and mood disorders? I didn't.

When eliminating sugar from your diet, be careful what artificial sweetener you chose. Splenda isn't the greatest choice because it has the potential of decreasing our good intestinal bacteria by 50% and cause weight gain (Murphree, 2014). Again the artificial sweetener recommended by functional medicine doctors is stevia Another issue we discussed was drinking enough water, which I was not very good at. So I also increased my water intake. That is vital to the healing process

process because it helps flush our body systems and aids in losing those fat cells that store inflammatory chemicals.

I was provided a booklet called *The Complete Patient Guidebook* published by Shape Re-Claimed. This book gave me specific directions as to what fruits and veggies I could eat as well as foods I had to stay away from. Again, I was also sent a personalized plan based on my food allergies and individual lab results. As a part of the program I purchased Dr Murphree sent me his book titled *Treating and Beating Fibromyalgia & Chronic Fatigue Syndrome*. I must say it opened up a whole new world of understanding for me as well as introduced me to some great information. Remember, knowledge is power. I highly recommend this book if you want more detailed information. I am merely scraping the tip of the iceberg when it comes to introducing you to the multiple ways you can help yourself. Here is a picture if you need it for a reference.

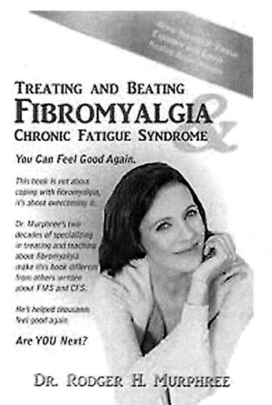

The other dietary issue I'd like to share that seems to be helping me is eating anti-inflammatory foods. I went on Google and looked up what foods fit into that category. I listed those foods in chapter five for you as well as resources, but it definitely was not an all-inclusive list.

Up to this point in time it has been 14 weeks since I started working with Dr. Murphree. Here is a list of the benefits I have experienced since I began:

1. I am sleeping 5-6 hours in a row if not more on most nights. I get a total of 8 hours of sleep on most nights.

2. I have eliminated the need for blood pressure pills.

3. I have eliminated Seroquel, a med with nasty side effects, pre-scribed to help me sleep.

4. I have eliminated the need to take a diuretic because of swelling I was experiencing as a side effect of some of my meds.

5. I have cut my gabapentin (Neurotonin) dose from 1800mg /day down to 900mg/day.

6. I am losing approximately 1/2 pound per day. I take drops manu-factured by Shape Re-Claimed prior to eating meals that actually helps eliminate fat cells.

Again, I cannot stress enough that each of us are slightly chemically different and what works for one person is not necessarily what will work best for another. I highly suggest you find a functional medicine doctor or someone who has had extended training in nutrition and natural supplements. Chaces are you will benefit from a holistic approach as opposed to just having medications prescribed for every symptom you are experiencing.

The supplements I am taking are advised specifically for me. Nevertheless, if you do research on some natural supplements I am sure you will find things you can safely use. The chart below includes a list of the supplements and the purpose for each of them.

| Supplement | Reason for use |
| --- | --- |
| Adrenal Cortex | Adrenal Insufficiency |
| Liver detox | Abnormal liver enzymes secondary to medications |
| L-Theanine | Relaxing effect |
| SAMe | Potent Pain reliever, anti-depressant, elevates mood |
| DHEA | Adrenal insufficiency: an adrenal steroid hormone converted to hormones that regulate fat and mineral metabolism, sexual and reproductive function, and energy level |
| Probiotic | Reduce growth of harmful bacteria/ promotes healthy digestive & immune system |
| Kinevace | Sleep |
| UltraPM Kinevace | Sleep |
| Melatonin | Sleep |
| Magnesium Maleate | Magnesium deficit, muscle spasms and cramps |
| Magnesium Citrate | Magnesium deficit, muscle spasms and cramps |
| Re-Claimed Shape drops | Helps with weight loss |
| 5-HTP | Turns into Serotonin helpful with: sleep, appetite, temperature, sexual behavior, and pain (I had to discontinue taking it), I had an allergic reaction to an herb in it |
| Vitamin Packet | It's important to supplement your nutrition with a good multi vitamin |
| Pentadolex | For migraines. I used to have migraines 2-3 times/week. I have only had 1 migraine in 2 ½ months. |
| L-Tryptophan | Turns into Serotonin |

## FIBRO IN THE SPOTLIGHT

As FM sufferers, we are no longer totally forgotten. There are multiple studies going on as to the cause and best way to treat fibro. Additionally, there are celebrities shining the spotlight on FM. I would like to mention just a few examples, and then give you some resources to investigate if you are interested in participating in a clinical trial.

There is an ongoing trial investigating the herpes simplex virus 1 (HSV-1) as a cause of fibromyalgia. The title of this article is "Big Antiviral Trial Could Usher in New Treatment Era for Fibromyalgia." The hypothesis is that the HSV-1 virus enters our system through the gut. I would like to mention that both doctors involved in this study propose their "treatment will work for chronic fatigue syndrome, irritable bowel syndrome, chronic pain, chronic headache, chronic neck pain, chronic back pain, chronic depression, chronic clinical anxiety disorder, post-traumatic stress disorder (PTSD), brain fog, cognitive dysfunction and chronic interstitial cystitis." **(http://www.prohealth.com/library/showarticle. cfm?libid=18809).**

I have come across some information that I find especially encouraging for those of us with FM. There is a Dr. Jarred Younger from Birmingham, Alabama who is working on establishing a research and clinical care center to specialize in FM, CFS, and Gulf war syndrome. Apparently he is already investigating and has found some highly probable underlying causes and promising treatments to relieve pain and fatigue, without side effects!

His research involves the immune system, special immune cells that defend the brain called microglia, and leptin which is a protein released by fat cells. According to Younger, leptin has the ability to cross over the protective blood brain barrier and activate or turn on the microglia cells when they are not supposed to be on. The result is pain, fatigue, depression, or interference with one's ability to think. However, Younger has yet to come up with a way to observe activation or inflammation in the human brain, because unfortunately there is no current way to observe this in humans. He is, however, looking into specialized brain scanning equipment that can measure certain chemicals and the temperature in the brain.

We have a strong advocate for the FM team. Not only does Dr. Younger believe that fibromyalgia exists and affects the body as a whole, he has made it his mission to figure out what is wrong and methods to treat FMS. His work is proclaimed to be cutting-edge and groundbreaking according to Dr. David McLain who is rheumatologist in Birmingham, Alabama. **(http://thehealthdisorder.com/uab-researcher-hoping-to-solve-mysteries-of-fibromyalgia-help-patients-break-free/)**

For those of you who are football fans, I am sure the name Dominique Easley who plays for the New England Patriots sounds familiar. Dominique has a sister named Destinee who was diagnosed with FM at age 12. She is about 17 years old now. He has a website **easleysawareness.com**, which tells his sister's story as well as his plans to promote awareness and education about FM. He has become an advocate for fibromyalgia and stated "What my plan is, is to raise enough money for women that can't really afford to come out — if Dr. Tad's treatments work — for women that can't really afford to come out here, to try to service them and (fund their trip) out here to do the treatments," **(Fibrotoday.com)**. Hopefully with his status in the National Football League, Dominique will bring more lots of attention and perhaps funds to promote research for a cure.

Lastly, it is my hope to personally invade the media with information that will make people, families, and medical professionals stand up and recognize that millions of people with similar symptoms are not crazy, hypochondriacs, or lunatics running around the United States and world. I had what I believe to be a practice audition to present my fibro information that I'd like to share with you.

Several years ago when I was still able to work, I took my nursing students to a nursing conference to give them a new experience. When I arrived, they asked if I was a teacher or student. I told them I was a nursing instructor. The lady checking me in suddenly smiled and said, "Oh my, thank the Lord. Your students told us you could help us out by being a guest speaker today." I looked around, laughed, and expected this to be a practical joke. It wasn't. I was told that a speaker called in sick, and they needed help. I looked at the agenda. The only possible topic I could speak to was fibromyalgia which happened to be the guest speaker who was ill. I hesitantly asked for 5 minutes to think about it.

To make a long story short, I was seated and the president of the Michigan Licensed Practical Nursing Association came and thanked me for agreeing to help, which I had not agreed to yet. I told her I would help, but could not speak to the power point presentation prepared by the speaker who was ill, but would just share my personal journey with fibro.

I was to be the second speaker. My teaching partner quickly gave me her I-pad so I could look up a brief history and jot down a few notes. Let me say, I did some serious praying prior to my brief preparation time. The first web site I looked at regarding history gave me chills. My prayer was answered. I found that the history is suspected to date back to the biblical days of Job. I jotted down the biblical scripture verse, a few other notes, and then a few personal things I had experienced.

Next thing I knew I was up in front of between 200-250 people talking about my complicated journey with fibromyalgia. I was told I only needed to speak for 15 minutes for them to get their accreditation, however, I ended up speaking 45 minutes. There were several questions, and it was one of the best spontaneous talks I had ever given. Afterwards, many people walked up to me and thanked me for putting a face with the name of a very complicated and mysterious illness they had no idea about. I was also told that it would certainly help them know how to be a better nurse to those with the illness.

After every professional conference they have the participants fill out an evaluation. I asked the conference coordinators if I could get feedback from my presentation. Approximately six months later, I received an e-mail that said I was the best presenter at the conference. I could hardly believe it, and laughed out loud. I am ready to spread the word about fibro, and believe I passed that audition with flying colors.

These are but a few of the new happenings that have brought FM into the limelight. Hopefully the doctors that verbalize that there is no such thing as fibro will be forced to believe it is real in light of the research and information that has been discovered and is forthcoming. I know I am extremely thankful for all the doctors and researchers who do believe FMS is real and who are dedicated to helping find an underlying cause, treatment, and perhaps a cure.

## CLINICAL TRIAL WEBSITES

### *Clinical Trial Info:*

1. https://www.clinicaltrials.gov/ct2/results?term=fibromyalgia&no_unk=Y&pg=1

2. Fibro Clinical Trials listed according to States: https://www.centerwatch.com/clinical-trials/listings/condition/218/fibromyalgia

3. http://www.nfra.net/opportunities.htm

4. http://patient.info/health/fibromyalgia-leaflet/clinical-trials

5. https://www.clinicaltrialsgps.com/clinical-trials-indications/fibromyalgia/

6. http://www.fmcpaware.org/clinical-trials2.html

# FUNCTIONAL MEDICINE DOCTORS

### *Fibromyalgia Doctors: Which one is best?*

http://www.myfibro.com/fibromyalgia-doctors

Friendly Fibro Doctors and Much More---National Fibromyalgia Association-websites

www.National FibromyalgiaandChronicPainAssociation.com

www.aolsearch.com/Physician+Directory

www.about.com/Fibromyalgia + Specialist

www.searchall.com/Doctors +Fibromyalgia

www.fibrocenter.com

www.myfibro.com/Fibromyalgia +Doctors

www.painfromfibromyalgia.com

www.fibrowellnesspeople.com

www.wedmed.com

http://www.womenshealth.gov/publications/our-publications/fact-sheet/fibromyalgia.html#j

### *Fibro Doctors:*

Kalliopi Nestor, MD

Board-certified: American Board of Physical Medicine & Rehabilitation

SPECIALIZES IN FIBROMYALGIA!

Office: 1001 East Second Street

Coudersport, PA 16915

Phone: 814.274.5320

DISTRICT OF COLUMBIA:

Dr. Sean Whelton, Department of Rheumatology

Georgetown University Hospital

Pasquerilla Health Center,

6th Floor 3800 ervoir Road. N.W.

Washington, D.C. 20007

202-444-6200 Main Phone and Patient Information

1-1-1471 X

1-1-1472

### INDIANA

Dr. Gregory Toothman

4015 Gateway Boulevard, Newburgh, IN 47630 (812) 858-9400

http://www.deaconess.com/DCBio/890


Dr. Anne Butsch: this clinic accepts low-income patients and Medicaid recipients

ECHO Community Healthcare

315 Mulberry Street Evansville, IN 47713 812-421-7489

http://www.echochc.org/

### ILLINOIS

Dr. Steven D. Diamond Primary Care Rockford, Illinois (815) 397-3337

http://diamondfmc.com/

### NEW YORK:

Dr. Elizabeth Reintz Rhuematology

Westchester County, New York

(914)723-8100

http://www.scarsdalemedical.com/


Dr. Joyce Reyes-Thomas Rhuematology

Westchester County, New York (914) 723-8100

http://www.scarsdalemedical.com/


## TENNESSEE

Dr. Lynn J. Williams Primary Care

Decherd, Tennessee (931) 962-0561

http://www.healthgrades.com/group-directory/tennessee-tn/decherd/j-lynn-williams-md-0009439?autosuggest=true


## VIRGINIA

Steven J. Maesstrello  Rhuematology

Richmond, Virginia

(804) 346-1551

http://www.healthgrades.com/physician/dr-steven-maestrello-x2gnd


## WISCONSIN

Dr. Jeffery B. Gorelick  Physiatrist Milwaukee,

Wisconsin (414) 771-2707

http://www.healthgrades.com/group-directory/wisconsin-wi/milwaukee/pain-rehabilitation-associates-8980bffd

# CHAPTER 7

# SOCIAL SECURITY DISABILITY AND FIBROMYALGIA

*Don't give up the fight, stand up for your rights*

*Bob Marley*

While it is not possible for me to tell you everything you need to know regarding disability, because it is a complicated process and the laws are always changing, it is possible that you can prepare yourself to the best of your ability before applying. The goal of this chapter is to educate you on how the process works, how to begin the process, the best way to file a claim, resources for you to use as reference if you do have to file your own paperwork, and just an overall idea as to what you can expect through this very complicated and sometimes frustrating process.

I'm not sure if you have heard as many horror stories about "Disability" as I have. Have you applied for disability and been denied? Are you afraid to even try to apply? Don't be afraid, but you must be informed! I have dedicated this chapter to help provide an overview and tips for those of you needing help to apply for Social Security Disability (SSDI) and Supplemental Security Income (SSI). Let me conclude this paragraph by stating I will be listing the web sites that I found this information on, at the end of the chapter.

Let's first distinguish the difference between SSI and SSDI. To be eligible for SSDI means you have worked a significant amount of time and paid into social security. There are classifications according to age, and they are as follows:

1.  If you are 31 or older you must have worked at least 10 years.

2.  Ages 24-31: you must have worked at least 7 years since you turned 21.

3.  Under the age of 24 means you must have worked at least a year and a half out of the past three years.

SSDI does not take into consideration your spouse's income or any investments you may have. But there is a limit on the amount of money you can earn while receiving disability. If you are well enough to work and earn more than $1,090 per month, then you are disqualified.

Let's discuss what SSI means. This income is for those individuals who haven't worked, or haven't worked enough to qualify for SSDI, for children with disabilities, and there is an income and asset limit for SSI because this program is specifically aimed at low income, elderly, or those who blind or incapacitated. Income restrictions are as follows:

1.  A single person: assets cannot exceed $2,000, and you cannot earn more than $733.00/month

2.  Married: assets cannot exceed $3,000, and your income cannot exceed $1,090 per month

After getting approved with my first application, which was a blessing, I called SSDI with some questions. They told me directly how fortunate

I was to be approved with my first application because most people get denied. Fortunately, I had a representative called "The Advocate Group" which was a service offered through my long term disability company. However, they are available for anyone to use, and they do not collect money unless they win your case.

My advice for anyone and everyone going through this process is, do NOT file the paperwork without a lawyer or representative, if possible. Here is a web site that will allow you to enter your zip code and connect with your lawyer in your area: http://www.disabilitysecrets.com/social_security_disability_fibromyalgia.html. There are attorneys that specialize in disability and often times they take a case and don't get paid unless you win the case. It is worth the time and hassle. I have heard so many nightmare stories about the multiple pages of paperwork and the multiple months that turn into years of waiting. So I strongly suggest you get legal representation if at all possible.

A big part of the reason people were not getting approved for FM is due to the fact that there was no "listing" or code of FM. So in 2012, the Social Security Administration (SSA) provided standards for all administrators, claims examiners, and judges to follow. It is said that these rules should help to increase the number of FM cases get approved.

## How SSA Views Fibromyalgia

It will be no big surprise for those of you with FM to hear that since FM is such a subjective condition, based on what the patient reports, as opposed to objective testing like x-rays, that FM was extremely misunderstood. However, since the new standards have been developed they have to view it differently.

There is a term called medically determinable impairment (MDI) which means that there must be medical evidence and not just patient reported symptoms of pain, fatigue, insomnia, foggy thinking, etc. The 2012 ruling gives instructions to all those involved in the process of denying or approving disability for FM must be based on the criteria set forth by the American College of Rheumatology (ACR). Additionally, the patient with widespread pain, especially in chest, neck, or back, must have been examined and had diagnostic labs and x-rays to rule out other medical conditions. In addition to that the patient must have one of the following:

1. At least 11 of 18 of the tender points as discussed in chapter 1.

   a.) The tender spots must occur on both sides of the body.

   b.) The tender spots must also occur above and below the waist.

2. The patient must also have six or more recurring incidents of the following FM symptoms:

   a.) Fatigue

   b.) Non-restorative sleep

   c.) Fibro fog: memory or thinking problems

   d.) Depression

   e.) Anxiety

   f.) Irritable bowel syndrome

   g.) Other possible acceptable symptoms:

3. muscle weakness

4. abdominal pain

5. Raynaud's syndrome

6. Seizures

7. Dizziness

In order to get started you will need to call your Social Security Administration Offices and schedule an interview. You can expect the interview to last approx. 90 minutes. This process can also be done online if you prefer. There is a multitude of information you will need in order to be ready for the interview. Additional information found at the following web site includes: common mistakes to avoid, what happens if your application is approved, denied, additional web sites when applying for disability. Keep in mind that once you have applied you will wait approximately six months for an answer. The aforementioned information can be found at **http://standinguptopots.org/livingwithpots/ disability.**

It's especially important to know that your doctor's notes will be scrutinized for evidence of pain, fatigue, and thinking problems. Thus your physician must be sure and have these notations in your medical file along with how long you have had these symptoms, how severe they are, how the symptoms affect your ability to function, what treatments you have tried and if they were helpful, and how long your doctor expects your condition to take place. Please note that the longer you have had your symptoms, the better your chances are **(disabilitysecrets.com)**.

So if your condition is found to qualify as a medically determinable impairment, guess what? The process has just begun. The next step that will be taken is for SSA to evaluate your residual functional capacity (RFC). What that simply means is that you will be assessed to see if you can perform different levels of work duties. You will be evaluated as to how long you can sit, how much you can lift, how long you can stand, how long you can focus, how long you can stand, walk, whether you need a daily nap, or to lie down because of fatigue or exhaustion, do you have to prop your feet up during the day, use heat and cold, run to the bathroom periodically because of irritable bowel syndrome? Do you have to use heat and cold for your pain throughout the day? Additionally, it is vital to be sure that the intensity of your pain and how it limits you during the day is documented. This is why I strongly recommend a daily journal. I know that with my memory impairment, I have a hard time remembering from one day to the next all my symptoms that I experience. I have included a blank copy at the end of this chapter of the types of questions you can expect to see and answer when going through this process. In regards to functional limitations, remember these are VITAL in demonstrating to SSA why you are unemployable.

If you are denied the first time, you should appeal with the help of a disability lawyer simply because they know the laws and are familiar with the process. They know the latest case laws and can help find mistakes made by the people who disapproved your case. It is also highly advised that if you have only seen your primary doctor at this point, then you request a specialist, more specifically a rheumatologist which will only help solidify your case. (**disabilitysecrets.com**).

Keep in mind that the following tips are essential to the process of applying for disability: 1.) Make sure you have fibromyalgia as a diagnosis in your medical files, 2.) Try to see a specialist preferably a rheumatologist or chronic pain doctor, 3.) A FM diagnosis by a mental health professional is not as acceptable because it is believed they misuse or overuse FM as a diagnosis. 4.) Find out what your medical records contain so you can get an idea of how strong your case is.

I also want to mention that the more medical conditions you have, the better your case stands to get approved. For example, not only do I have fibromyalgia, but I was diagnosed with rheumatoid arthritis, adrenal insufficiency, steroid induced diabetes, severe decompensation as documented by a physical therapist; which leads me to an additional important point. The more specialists and medical documentation you have, the stronger your case is, which makes sense

Since chronic pain is not an acceptable diagnosis, I thought I would share with you some of the acceptable diagnoses I found which include: inflammatory arthritis, neurological disorders, somatoform disorders (mental illness causing physical symptoms including pain), back injury, chronic renal disease, and inflammatory bowel disease to name a few. Here is a web site that will give you 200+ listings, if you are interested: **http://www.disability-benefits-help.org/disabling-conditions.**

As a registered nurse one of the things I have been complimented on by many colleagues, is my ability to document very well. I have a suggestion regarding documentation of your symptoms that you are suffering from. My system seems to be effective because every time Met Life reviews my case every 3-4 months, I have no problems.

## SUGGESTIONS FOR DOCUMENTATION

My technique is very simple. I started at the top of my head and went to my feet and listed my symptoms. Additionally, I listed how the symptoms interfered with my life and daily abilities to function. One of the most important factors, in my opinion as a nurse, is to be very descriptive as to how your symptoms affect your safety. For example, my cognitive issues were so bad that it affected my judgement and ability to process information so I refused to drive because I did not feel safe. I was totally backed up by my physician who said I should not be driving. You will see more examples below as I share how I documented my problems. Feel free to use my format as a guide, but please remember to use your own symptoms and be completely honest when filling out forms. Below this documentation is a head to toe documentation tool if you care to use it to be a bit more organized.

Below is a sample of my personal list of signs and symptoms that I used to communicate with my physician and disability company—**and** the problems they cause me with my everyday life, ability to function, or not function. It is imperative that when you list your problems that you include what type of issue it interferes with in your everyday life abilities—I cannot stress that enough. You must communicate this with your physician so he/she can understand your issues.

Suggestion—I started from head to toe and just listed everything I could think of that was wrong with me and how I felt—it seemed to help me to have some type of system. Then I went back and listed why and how the ailment limited my ability to function. **BE VERY DESCRIPTIVE and be sure to include SAFETY ISSUES as well.**

Also—please see information below which contains info regarding PHYSICIAN DOCUMENTATION that is VITAL for you to know.

### Head to toe S/S:

» LOTS OF PAIN-generalized in muscles and joints, upper and lower back has a lot of pain-

» Conditions that exacerbate breathing- Humidity, certain scents, physically doing too much

» Blurred vision-been informed by endocrinologist to make an eye appointment

» Diabetes type 2- has caused permanent damage to patients one and only kidney- Kidney doctor consulted due to micro-albumin being >1000. Normal range 0-30

» Double vision at times- affects safety and ability to read

» Headaches: interferes with my ability to think clearly

» Migraines- approx. once monthly- causes me to be bedbound

» Foggy Brain-confusion

» Stuttering- cannot get the right words out

» Dizziness- safety issue, can easily lose balance

» Unable to tolerate bright light and loud sounds

» Disconnection from people and life

» Easily irritated

» Unable to tolerate bright light and loud sounds

» Inability at times to process what others are saying

» **Having a hard time communicating thoughts and comprehending new ones**

» Depression

» Not sleeping well

» **Require naps almost daily r/t fatigue**

» Pain is waking me up at night- (Fibro pain)

» Ringing in ears - makes it hard to hear

» Loss of balance at times- endangering my safety. I have fallen many times.

» Swelling of ankles, feet, and lower legs

» **\*\*\*DAILY Fatigue: this is a huge problem for patient because it interferes with my ability daily living abilities. I often don't get dressed because it's too painful and tiring.**

» Shortness of breath with mild to moderate activity- multiple rest periods required

» Red sunburn skin rash-located mostly on my arms and chest: there are times when I feel like I am going to pass out. I feel extremely weak, short of breath and lightheaded. I have several of these spells that come and go---no certain pattern. This puts me in my bed and I cannot function. These symptoms are associated with this rash

» Body Aches throughout back and arms, settling in arm joints, legs. Ankles, toes; I often take 2 naps a day about an hour each. Unable to sit for longer than 30 minutes.

» Muscle Spasms in any part of my body at any time- usually in hands and feet

» Muscle weakness- some falls- Latest fall _____- Damage caused: dislocated my sacroiliac joint which required seeing a chiropractor 3 times a week for 2 week. Restricted to NO Physical therapy for 4 weeks.

» Poor balance

» Skin discoloration –bruise like areas that bleed easily - (steroid side effect-it makes skin very thin)

» Constipation/Diarrhea-Irritable bowel syndrome

### *Physical limitations;*

1. Informed by Dr. NOT to drive.

2. Activities of daily living:

   a.) Shower chair because I get Short of breath trying to take a shower without it. This has improved somewhat over the past few months. The shortness of breath is not as severe as it was. I need help sometimes getting out of the shower due to loss of balance.

   b.) Dressing: Pt can do about 80% when it comes to getting dressed. Still need help sometimes when it comes to bra, shoes and sock. If too fatigued and in pain-there are days she doesn't bother getting dressed and stays in Pajamas.

   c.) Household chores: Patient is able to do light household chores-but states she must "pace herself." She can load the dishwasher and wipe kitchen cupboards-but then has to rest. (or) if you are unable to do chores state it.

      » Vacuums approx. twice weekly-which does cause mild SOB-has a 10 year old daughter that helps.

      » Pt states she has a house cleaner coming in 1X/mo to help.

   d.) Husband does 80% of the cooking.

   e.) Able to make simple foods to eat; Grilled cheese, fresh fruit, makes a salad.

f.) Who cares for Children-She goes to daycare once a week, sometimes she goes to friends' house for the day, she is pretty self-sufficient-makes her own meals- helps with household chores. Husband occasionally takes a day off to stay home with daughter.

3. (Anticipated question) **How often does patient leave the house and where does she go?**

a.) Pt states she leaves the house 1-2 times a month. States she does use an amigo when she goes to the store (Wal-Mart) to pick up odds and ends needed in the household-she has to have someone for transportation. On rare occasions, she will go out to breakfast with family.

b.) Every 3 months she goes to get her hair cut- needs transportation to get there.

c.) Leaves house for doctors' appointments----husband, mom, step- dad, or friends drive her.

d.) Pt states she is able to go out into yard-when humidity is not high. Pt states she got short of breath and very tired after this activity.

e.) Able to ride their riding lawn mower at approx. 30 minute intervals- needs to rest after that-states their yard is uneven, bumpy, and her arms and shoulders are in pain after mowing 30 minutes.

4. (Anticipated question) **What does a normal day consist of for the patient?**

a.) Waking up at around 4am every morning – mornings are very hard- lots of pain and very stiff. It takes 2-4 hours for this to diminish, but it never goes away.

b.) Pt states she tries to walk 5 minutes on treadmill every am, performs arm exercises with light arm weights, and also leg exercises with leg weights. It has been suggested by Physical therapy for patient to do planned exercises in spurts t/o the day and NOT all at one time because of the severe deconditioning.

c.) Social: Patient states she plays games on computer, reads (although it's hard because of blurry vision), writes in her journal, and spends lots of devotional time with God.

d.) Often goes back to bed at 10-11 am to rest.

e.) Gets up for lunch.

f.) Goes back to bed for a nap.

g.) Gets up and tries to exercise more with arm and leg weights.

h.) Eats dinner.

i.) Plays computer games/Facebook/researches landscaping ideas on Pinterest.

j.) To bed and watches movie with daughter.

5. Current medical conditions pt is being treated for:

    a.) Cushing's Syndrome r/t long term use of prednisone

    b.) Adrenal insufficiency, inability to wean prednisone, Pts body addicted to prednisone-going through withdrawal.

    c.) Restrictive lung disease- occasionally uses rescue inhaler (2xweek- and nebulizer if needed- approx. once weekly)

    d.) Fibromyalgia

    e.) Diabetes (steroid induced)- Diagnose 1/21/14

    f.) Anxiety

    g.) Vitamin D Deficiency,

    h.) Intermittent Depression,

    i.) GERD,

    j.) Thrush-intermittently-in mouth and throat-have med

    k.) Yeast infection under breasts

l.)  Intermittent sunburn type rash on face, arms, and chest

m.) Sleep Apnea: on c-pap since Jan 6, 2014

n.)  Restless leg syndrome

***Other conditions pt is being treated for:***

» CKD (chronic kidney disease) stage 2-3

» Meniere's disease-especially with weather changes-Pt gets dizzy and requires medication

» Insomnia

» PVC's (premature ventricular contractions) with low K+

» Hypoxia- with exertion

» Anemia- very low iron, low hgb

## HEAD TO TOE DOCUMENTATION TOOL

| Pain/ Problem | How long have I had the problem? | How it affects my ability to function | Meds or treatments attempted | What has been effective |
|---|---|---|---|---|
| | | | | |
| | | | | |
| | | | | |
| | | | | |

Another very important piece of information you need to be aware of is documenting every single physician you have seen along with their specialty and contact info. I am going to give you an example of my ongoing documentation of physicians I have seen over the last six years. I will not give you the complete list, because I am up to having seen around 50 doctors. My list includes four trips to Mayo Clinic and Cleveland clinic where I saw multiple doctors, but don't panic. I will only provide you with one example. Speaking of doctors, I want to engrain this into your brain. If you see a doctor and they tell you there is no such thing as fibro or that it's all in your head, RUN the other way and find a new doctor.

Dr. Christian Nasr, MD, FACP, FACE, ECNU- Endocrinology & Metabolism Institute, Thryoid Center Co-director

9500 Euclid Avenue/F20

Cleveland Ohio, 44195

Ph: 216-445-1788

Fax: 216-445-1656

Date of treatment: 4/16/14

Reason for visit: Life threatening Iatrogenic Cushing's Syndrome, adrenal insufficiency/steroid induced adrenal suppression, Thyroid problem, Significant morbidity from prednisone: skin, muscles, diabetes, mental functioning, Tachycardia

## ADDITIONAL IMPORTANT INFORMATION

Additional advice regarding this process and documentation includes: keeping an ongoing list of all the medications you are on, have tried, and whether they were effective for you or not. I didn't do a very good job of this because my meds were changing too quickly and my brain just could not keep up with everything that was going on. I was in and out of the hospital so many times and I truly lost track. You could make a chart like the one I have above, but just make it apply to your meds.

Be aware that you may also be asked to provide documentation as to what a day in the life of you, looks like. Here is a sample of what I mean.

***Daily Routine:*** Times are approximate and activities may vary a bit according to the day or whether I am going to physical therapy or aqua therapy 2x/weekly, have a doctor's appointment, or stay home; able to let our dog in/out throughout the day

**3am-4am:** Awake with steroid withdrawal, shaky inside and out, pain 4/10 all over but especially in fingers, toes, lower back, arms and legs

**4am-5am:** awake again- restless sleep

**6am-7am:** Awake and get up for the day

For the next 90 minutes- make & drink coffee, eat breakfast (yogurt or cereal), brush teeth, watch Christian TV, read my bible, read daily devotionals(in a book or on my computer), and walk on treadmill x 15 minutes (if it is not a physical therapy day), take Morning Meds

**9:30am:** Rest/Meditate

**10:00am-** check blood sugar

**10am-11:30am-** a few light household chores- varies from day to day-perhaps vacuum 2-3x/week, load dishwasher then put dishes away, dust once weekly, sit-check e-mails to rest/ write a letter or send emails to friends, eat a piece of fruit for a snack, perhaps write in my journal

**11:30am -** rest/meditate

**11:45am-1:30pm:** eat lunch (protein bar, cottage cheese with pineapple or something that takes little preparation), walk on treadmill 15 minutes, watch Joyce Meyer, listen to music or read for a little while, perhaps fold some laundry & put it away if my husband has washed and dried it and left it in our bedroom

**Between 1pm and 3pm:** I take a nap for approx. 20-30 minutes

**Upon awaking @ approx. 2pm-4pm:** I begin prepare dinner, I may put chicken breasts in the oven to bake, or make hamburger patties, nothing too elaborate, however, if I make a crock pot dinner-I would have put in in first thing in the am, watch for my daughter get off the bus at 3:00-unless she has after school activities, if that's the case-her dad picks her up, maybe spend some time on face book or play computer games for approx. 30-40 min, use my arm weights for 10-15 min, leg lifts and ankle circles for physical therapy exercises

**4pm:** relax/meditate for 10-20 min

**4:30pm-6pm:** eat dinner with my family, help my family clear table and dishes from dinner, walk on treadmill x 15 minutes, and spend time talking with my daughter about her day at school. Call or text a few friends, write a letter, read a little more, use my arm weights for 10-15 min, leg lifts and ankle circles for physical therapy exercises

**6pm-** relax/meditate for 10-20 minutes

**6:30pm-7:30pm:** Maybe load the dishwasher

**730pm-9pm:** start getting ready for bed, brush teeth, snuggle with daughter and watch TV or a movie, nightly snack-usually a bowl of cereal then take my nightly medications, perhaps write in my journal,

Depending on how tired I am I will go to bed between 9-10. I usually lie in bed and read approx. 30 minutes (my eyes still get tired and vision blurry after approx. 30 minutes-likely steroid related), or just lay in bed and relax and pray

After going to sleep I can only stay asleep for three to four hours at the most. After that I experience a very restless night including waking up on multiple occasions. I have recently started trying to take Melatonin in an effort to restore a regular sleeping pattern. It's too early to have noticed a difference yet. I do have sleep apnea and use my C-pap every night. I have noticed that makes a bit of a difference in how much I feel rested (as compared to how I felt before I started using it).

This is such a big process and so much to remember, but you will be guided by the paperwork they send you to fill out. I continue learning new things all the time. For example, just this past November 2015, I learned that I had been on disability for two years which means you automatically qualify for Medicare. Now here is something I never thought I would be dealing with: Medicare at the age of 49.

I'd like to bring something to your attention at this time. If you did not read Monica Mullens testimonial in the front of the book, now would be a good time to go back and read it. She contacted me regarding help in applying for disability. I supplied her with the information, resources, and web sites I have provided within this chapter, and she applied without any legal representation. Within three months she was approved. She could not thank me enough for supplying the info she needed to make this happen. So this info has been tried and true, even if for only one person so far. I am so thankful that I could be of help, and so is Monica.

I'd like to conclude this chapter by saying this can obviously be an overwhelming process to have to go through. That's why it is best to have legal help if possible. To try and condense this information as much as possible, I'd like to re-iterate a few very important pieces of documentation that you need to start keeping track of right now:

1. Keeping track of all your symptoms in a journal or log.

2. Be sure your doctor's documentation reflects your symptoms which includes the diagnosis of fibromyalgia and any other medical conditions.

3. Keep track of all your doctors and specialists you see along with the documented information as listed above in my example,

4. Be prepared to provide documentation of what your daily routine looks like.

5. Keep any and all documentation if you go into the hospital, have physical therapy, or any other medical therapies you attempt.

6. Ask for a copy of all your labs or diagnostics to be sent to you when results become available.

## RESOURCES

1. Applying for Disability : http://standinguptopots.org/livingwithpots/disability

2. Social Security Disability (SSDI & SSI) for Fibromyalgia: http://www.disabilitysecrets.com/resources/social-security-disability-ssdi-ssi-fibromyalgia.htm

3. Contacting Social Security: 1-800-772-1213, or www.socialsecurity.gov

# CHAPTER 8

---

# QUICK REFERENCE Q&A'S

*"As long as you're alive, keep learning and laughing"*

*~Kelly Hemingway~*

It is my sincere hope that I have been able to help those of you who suffer from FMS, chronic illness, or a chronic pain condition with some tools to help you cope and deal with your day to day obligations. My wish is also that I was able to help your family understand and bear the difficult times, but more than anything, I hope that I have made the point that you do not have to choose to let FM become your identity. There are so many different ways we can help ourselves. No, FM is not curable. But there is a life out there that you can have, chose to live it! Don't let fibro be your identity. Be the person who gets up every day and kicks its butt.

I am dedicating this last chapter as a question and answer forum, as well as an informational medium. Perhaps you have a new diagnosis, if so this chapter will hopefully provide you with some instant

---

information. Even if you have been dealing with chronic illness and pain for years, you may find enlightening information. I will close the chapter on a positive and uplifting note by sharing some more fibro fog stories that could really apply to anyone and everyone because we all do crazy things. However, it just seems that those of us with fibro, it's more than an everyday occurrence, it's an every hour occurrence sometimes. Lastly, I will provide more references for support groups and places you can attain more information.

1. **What is fibromyalgia?**

   A chronic pain disorder, related to arthritis, but it does not cause inflammation.

2. **What is the cause of Fibro?**

   There is no known cause, but multiple theories.

3. **What are the most common signs of fibromyalgia?**

   » Chronic widespread, persistent pain (stabbing, throbbing, aching, twitching)

   » Fatigue

   » Problems sleeping

   » According to the National Fibromyalgia Association: Possible associated conditions include but not limited to: "irritable bowel and bladder, headaches and migraines, restless legs syndrome, impaired memory and concentration, skin sensitivities and rashes, dry eyes and mouth, anxiety, depression, ringing in the ears, dizziness, vision problems, Raynaud's Syndrome, neurological symptoms, and impaired coordination."

   » 90% of fibro patients have jaw or facial tenderness that can produce jaw pain (http://www.myfibro.com/fibromyalgia-statistics)

4. **Who does fibro affect the most?**

80-90% are women. However men and children can get it also. (nih.org)

**5. How many people have FM?**

Approximately 5 million Americans and the diagnosis usually occur in middle adult hood.

**6. What is a fibro flare?**

It occurs when there is an exacerbation or worsening of your fibro symptoms. It can be mild or as severe as making you want to stay in bed.

**7. What are the major causes of a fibro flare?**

» Emotional Distress

» Weather changes

» Sleeping problems

» strenuous activity

» Mental Stress

» Worrying

» Traveling in a car

» Family fights

» Physical injuries

» Physical inactivity

(http://www.myfibro.com/fibromyalgia-statistics)

**8. What is fibro fog?**

Trouble with concentration, memory, and confusion.

**9. What's the best doctor to diagnose and treat FM?**

Rheumatologist, neurologist, or a doctor familiar with FM.

**10. Does every FM patient have the same symptoms?**

No, in fact it is said that no two FM patients are alike.

**11. How much of a problem is sleep for the FM patient?**

Approximately 90% of patients with FM have sleep disorders.

**12. Why is it so hard for doctors to diagnose FM?**

FM has symptoms that mimic many other conditions.

**13. Is it possible to have FM and CFS?**

Yes, in fact up to 70% of FM patients exhibit and fulfil criteria for CFS. (uptodate.com)

**14. Is Fibro hereditary?**

According to Mayo Clinic there does appear to be some genetic markers in the DNA, thus leading researchers to believe it may run in families.

**15. What can I do to help my FM symptoms?**

Medication, natural supplements, exercise, relaxation, stress-reduction are but a few things you can do. (Mayoclinic.org)

**16. What is some good advice for FM patients to remember?**

a.) It's ok to say no.

b.) Listen to what your body is telling you.

c.) Nutrition can make a difference.

d.) Find positive coping skills to handle stress.

e.) Think holistically: do things that will benefit your mind, body, and soul.

**17. What are the risk factors for FM?**

Being a woman, family history, and having a rheumatic disease. (mayoclinic.org)

**18. Is FM progressive?**

It depends on who you ask. Some research says no it is not, some research says yes it is. Most importantly people suffering from it say they have noticed it can get worse over time.

**19. What is a good way to help my family and friends understand how I feel with having FM?**

Have them listen and watch The Spoon Theory video.

https://www.youtube.com/watch?v=jn5lBsm49Rk

Tell them it feels like you have the flu every day of your life in addition to all over pain in your body that compares to low back pain. I read an article that said many people can identify with how painful and limiting back pain can be, so this might be one way to help people understand how limited you are.

**20.  Do my thoughts really affect how I physically feel?**

YES! There is a mind body connection and studies have been done that prove optimism reduces stress-induced inflammation and stress hormones.

**21. What is the best way to help my muscle pain?**

EPSOM SALT SOAKS and Magnesium Supplements.

Many fibro sufferers have a magnesium deficiency, so adding a supplement is usually a good idea. You should consult with a physician first before adding any supplements because you will likely need labs drawn. PLUS there are many different sources of magnesium supplements, some are better than others depending on what other health conditions you suffer from.

**22. What are some easy ways to raise my serotonin levels?**

Eating bananas, oats, almonds, walnuts, leafy green vegetables, drinking plenty of water, cayenne peppers, chocolate (high in magnesium), or a smoothie made from green vegetables.

**23. Is it true that negative emotions can harm your body?**

YES! Anger can weaken the liver and raise your blood pressure

Grief- weakens the lungs

Worry- weakens the stomach

Stress- weakens the heart, brain and immune system

Fear- weakens the kidneys

(this is just a brief list-there are many other damaging effects of negative feelings)

**24. What are some things I should keep handy for my fibro tool-kit?**

» Muscle creams (Emu oil, Tiger balm)

» Massage utensils

» A Rice bag or heating pad

» Warm fuzzy socks or slippers

» Dark Chocolate (remember it's a mood booster and helps produce serotonin)

» Lotion for dry skin

» Extra blankets and pillows in your living room or family room

## ADVICE/COMMENTS FROM FIBRO FOLKS

*You kind of just have to follow your bodies lead...not what your brain is telling you.*

*I wish I would have known how fibro affects so many parts of the body.*

*I wish I would have known how much my life would change.*

*You are going to want to give up. DON'T!*

*Don't keep your feelings bottled up.*

*Be prepared for doctors or medical personnel to not believe you or tell you it's all in your head.*

*Physical exercise really does help, just do what you can, everyone is different*

*If you have a doctor that does not believe fibro is real, find a new one.*

*Never give up, stand your ground.*

## FIBRO FOG FUNNIES

Yes we can be crazy, but we have to learn to laugh it off!

*Today I cautiously snuck up on and killed a piece of fuzz!*

*Sprayed my face with makeup brush cleaner instead of spray to set makeup.*

*Last week I was needing to text my son, I looked everywhere, that darn phone, finally had my husband call it and it was in my hand the whole time!*

*I put the entire coffee pot in the fridge today then asked my boyfriend, "What happened to the coffee pot? It's not where it should be." He said, "Well it couldn't have gone far." And there it was in the fridge.*

*So I've traveled to see my rheumatologist 40 mins in car only to get there and find out I'm a day early!!!! Fibro fog at its best.*

*I tried to fry some french fries in Karo (corn syrup).*

*I have put milk in the cupboard and cereal in the refrigerator.*

*My hubby poured his glass of water into the toaster instead of the sink.*

*I put the milk in the cupboard instead of the fridge and wondered where the milk was the next day when I went to grab a glass. Yuck! Spoiled milk.*

*Driving and totally forget where I'm going!!!! My son has to remind me!!!*

*I couldn't find my purse anywhere, turned up in the freezer.*

*Just a couple of weeks ago, I punched my phone number in to the microwave!*

*I went to the police station this am to file a report and the cop asked me for my license. I started digging through my purse and couldn't find it. So this cop says to me, "So you're telling me you are driving without a license?" I said, "I guess I am."*

*I'm 38 years old and forgetting things...last weekend left the oven on all night, this week put a block of cheese in the freezer and blamed my husband for eating it, then I couldn't remember my own address I had to text my husband at work to ask what unit # we live in.*

In conclusion, there should be no shred of doubt that fibro is real, Not only does it qualify as a chronic illness causing physical, mental, emotional, and spiritual issues for the sufferer, but the family unit as a whole is also affected. Keeping an open line of communication will likely empower and strengthen the relationships between the person suffering from chronic illness and their loved ones as well as their medical health care team.

It is vital that you or your family member who lives with chronic pain to take control of and educate yourself as to what the best treatment is for you. Many times a combination of traditional, natural supplements and alternative methods of treatments are most effective. The most important thing for you to remember is that you don't have to settle for the words "You'll have to learn to live with the pain." There are options.

Fibromyalgia has finally been given its own medical code and recognized as a real illness. It's also starting to get more and more attention with clinical trials, celebrities, and a blood test to "rule-in" as opposed to having fibromyalgia being ruled out and using us as a medical pin cushion. If fibro has affected your quality of life to the point where you aren't able to work, as it has me at this point in my life, please know that disability is an option. Again, empower yourself with information and get an advocate or lawyer if you can. If not, there are plenty of web sites online to help you in addition to the ones I have also provided. We have not made the decision to have fibro or a chronic illness, but surrounding that "non-choice" are a million other choices we can make (paraphrased from a quote from Michael J. Fox). Remember, you have fibro, but it doesn't have to have you!

# RESOURCES

*Worldwide Information about Fibro:*

http://www.rightdiagnosis.com/f/fibromyalgia/stats-country.
htm#extrapwarning

*National Fibromyalgia and Chronic Pain Association:*

http://www.fmcpaware.org/fibromyalgia/prevalence.html

*Support for Fibro and Chronic Fatigue:*

http://www.myfibro.com/fibromyalgia-statistics

*Tools to help fibro symptoms:*

http://wp.me/p6Brx9-d1

Mayo Clinic has a Fibro Education Center that you can call and request educational resources for free: 507-248-8140

» **Arthritis Foundation**
   **Phone:** 800-283-7800

» **National Fibromyalgia Association**
   **Phone:** 714-921-0150

» **National Fibromyalgia Partnership, Inc.**
   **Phone:** 866-725-4404

» **National Institute of Arthritis and Musculoskeletal and Skin Diseases**
   **Phone:** 877-226-4267

If you need more information about available resources in your language or another language, please visit our website or contact the NIAMS Information Clearinghouse at **NIAMSinfo@mail.nih.gov.**

### *Links to Other Fibromyalgia Resources*

Here are a number of online fibromyalgia resources you may want to take time to explore.

Association and Community Websites

Medical Websites

Government Websites

Pfizer FM Resources

### *Association and Community Websites*

American Chronic Pain Association

American Fibromyalgia Syndrome Association (AFSA)

Fibromyalgia Network

HealthyWomen

National Fibromyalgia Research Association (**NFRA**)

National Women's Health Resource Center

National Fibromyalgia and Chronic Pain Association (NFMCPA)

American Association of Nurse Practitioners (AANP)

### *Medical Websites*

American College of Rheumatology

familydoctor.org (a website run by the American Academy of Family Physicians [AAFP], a national medical organization representing family physicians, family practice residents, and medical students)

researchers of Mayo Clinic) **MayoClinic.com** (a website offering medical information from the physicians, scientists, and

WebMD (a health information site with medical news, features, reference material, and online community programs)

## *Government Websites*

Medline Plus (Health information from the National Library of Medicine. Includes medical journal articles, information about drugs, and more)

National Institute of Arthritis and Musculoskeletal and Skin Diseases (NIAMS)

## *Pfizer FM Resources*

FibroCenter.com Facebook Page

Fibroknowledge.com (a website where health care professionals can learn more about fibromyalgia diagnosis and clinical studies)

The FibroCollaborative Roadmap for Change: A Call to Action for Fibromyalgia

https://www.facebook.com/FibroCenter/

https://www.fibrocenter.com/sites/g/files/g10027391/f/201510/ PBP773103_%23FibroTalk%20Webchat%203%20FOR%203%20Tool_FINAL. PDF

## *Sites for fibromyalgia in Canada*

» Canada's health network for women:

http://www.cwhn.ca/node/40784

» My health Alberta

https://myhealth.alberta.ca/Alberta/Pages/living-with-fibromyalgia.aspx

» Chronic pain association:

http://chronicpaincanada.com/support/contacts

*Fibromyalgia Support Groups - England, Ireland, Scotland and Wales.*

http://www.fibromyalgia-support.net/support/index.html

## RESOURCES

1. Burckhardt CS, Goldenberg D, Crofford L, et al. Guideline for the Management of Fibromyalgia Syndrome Pain in Adults and Children. APS Clinical Practice Guidelines Series, No.4. Glenview, Ill: American Pain Society; 2005.

2. Arnold, L, Clauw, D, McCarberg, B. Improving the Recognition and Diagnosis of Fibromyalgia. Mayo Clin Proc. 2011; 86(5):457-464.

3. National Institute of Arthritis and Musculoskeletal and Skin Diseases. Questions and Answers about Fibromyalgia. Available at: http://www.niams.nih.gov/Health_Info/Fibromyalgia/default.asp. Accessed April 10, 2012.

4. Arnold, L, Hudson, J, Hess, E, Ware, A, Fritz, D, Auchenbach, M, Starck, L, Keck, P. Family study of fibromyalgia. Arthritis & Rheumatism. 2004 March;50(3):944-952.

5. The Fibrocollaborative Roadmap for Change. 2009. Available at: http://www.npwh.org/files/public/FibroCollaborative%20Roadmap%20(2).pdf

6. Mayo Clinic. Fibromyalgia: Risk Factors. Available at: http://www.mayoclinic.com/health/fibromyalgia/DS00079/DSECTION=risk-factors. Accessed April 10, 2012.

7. Synovate. [data]. Chronic Pain Consumer Survey. March 2011.

8. Henriksson KG. Fibromyalgia — from syndrome to disease. Overview of pathogenetic mechanisms. J Rehabil Med. 2003;41(suppl):89-94.

9. Wolfe, F, Ross, K, Anderson, J, Russell, J, Hebert, L. The prevalence and characteristics of fibromyalgia in the general population. Arthritis & Rheumatism. 1995 Jan;38:19-28.

10. ACPA. Fibromyalgia. Available at: www.theacpa.org/conditionDetail.aspx?id=1. Accessed April 10, 2012.

11. Wolfe, F, Smythe, H, Yunus, M, et al. The american college of rheumatology 1990 criteria for the classification of fibromyalgia. Arthritis and Rheumatism. 1990 Feb;33(2):160-172.

12. Wolfe, F, Clauw, D, Fitzcharles, MA, et al. The american college of rheumatology preliminary diagnostic criteria for fibromyalgia and measurement of symptom severity. Arthritis Care & Research. 2010 May;62(5):600-610.

13. Pfizer Market Research, Data on File. 2010.

14. Goldenberg, D, Burckhardt, C, Crofford, L. Management of fibromyalgia syndrome. Journal of the American Medical Association. 2004;292(19):2388-2395.

15. Inanici F, Yunus MB. History of fibromyalgia: past to present. Curr Pain Headach Rep. 2004 Oct;8(5):369-78.

16. Fibrocenter. History of fibromyalgia. Available at: https://fibrocenter.pfizer.edrupalgardens.com/fibromyalgia-disease. Accessed April 10, 2012.

17. American Pain Foundation. About APF. Available at: http://www. painfoundation.org/about/. Accessed April 10, 2012.

18. National Fibromyalgia Association. About the national fibromyalgia association. Available at: http://fmaware.org/site/PageServerc91e. html?pagename=about_nfa. Accessed April 10, 2012.

19. ACPA. September is Pain Awareness Month. Available at: www. theacpa.org/69/Septemberispainawarenessmonth.aspx. Accessed April 10, 2012.

20. Amazon. The arthritis foundation's guide to good living with fibromyalgia. Available at: http://www.amazon.com/Arthritis-Foundations-Guide-Living-Fibromyalgia/dp/0912423269. Accessed April 10, 2012.

21. Food and Drug Administration. FDA approves first drug for treating fibromyalgia. Available at: http://www.fda.gov/NewsEvents/Newsroom/PressAnnouncements/2007/ucm108936.htm. Accessed April 10, 2012.

22. Lilly. Corporate Press Release. Available at: http://newsroom.lilly.com/ releasedetail.cfm?releaseid=316740. Accessed April 17, 2012.

23. Forest Laboratories / Cypress Bioscience. Corporate Press Release. Available at: http://news.frx.com/press-release/product-news. Accessed April 23, 2012.

24. HealthyWomen. Women and men face off: Who can stand the pain? Available at: http://www.healthywomen.org/content/press-release/women-and-men-face-who-can-stand-pain-0?context=press-release/2009&context_title=press%20releases&context_description. Accessed April 11, 2012.

25. NFMCPA. National Fibromyalgia & Chronic Pain Association Releases Inaugural Edition of Fibromyalgia & Chronic Pain LIFE(TM)

Magazine. Available at: http://www.prweb.com/releases/2011/9/pr-web8762005.htm. Accessed April 11, 2012.

26. Pfizer Market Research, Data on File. 2011.

27. Eli Lilly. Know Fibro Initiative Commemorates National Pain Awareness Month. Available at: http://newsroom.lilly.com/releasedetail.cfm?releaseid=407413. Accessed April 18, 2012.

28. HealthyWomen. Delay in Diagnosis Significantly Impacts Lives of Patients with Fibromyalgia, New Survey Reports. Available at: http://www.healthywomen.org/content/press-release/delay-diagnosis-significantly-impacts-lives-patients-fibromyalgia-new-survey-r. Accessed April 18, 2012.

# ABOUT THE AUTHOR

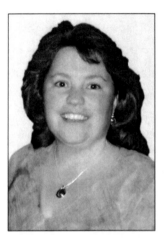

I reside in the Great Lake State of Michigan with a total of 4 of his, hers, and our children ranging in ages from 12 to 30 years old. I have been a registered nurse for 22 years. I graduated from the University of Michigan with my Bachelors in nursing and from Walden University with my Masters in Nursing with Specialization in Education. I have had the honor of speaking at and educating others about teaching strategies at several state nursing conferences as well as share my fibromyalgia journey at a Licensed Practical Nursing state conference

My nursing experience includes medical surgical nursing, case management/discharge planning, and I have worked a cardiac intensive care unit nurse. After many years of hospital nursing I became the lead nursing instructor for the Licensed Practical Nursing program at a community college, educating both in the classroom and a clinical setting, until I was struck by a life threatening allergic reaction. My health plummeted and I lost my career as a result of multiple health conditions including fibromyalgia.

My goal is to educate, empower, and legitimize fibromyalgia as a diagnosis. My mission: to support, educate and advocate. That is why I am a member of an online fibro support group as one of the leaders who helps educate and uplift all members. Additionally, I share my journey with a functional medicine doctor, Dr Murphree, who is helping me convert to natural supplements for treatments. After educating myself about this illness, I want to proclaim that you do not have to accept the statement "You will just have to learn to live with this."

Although I have accepted my diagnosis of fibromyalgia, I have consciously decided to not let it steal my life. I hope and pray you will do the same. Blessings to you all.